IMAGERY-BASED COGNITIVE THERAPY
FOR BIPOLAR DISORDER AND MOOD INSTABILITY

Imagery-Based Cognitive Therapy for Bipolar Disorder and Mood Instability

Emily A. Holmes
Susie A. Hales
Kerry Young
Martina Di Simplicio

Foreword by Gillian Butler

Afterword by Guy Goodwin

THE GUILFORD PRESS
New York   London

Copyright © 2019 The Guilford Press
A Division of Guilford Publications, Inc.
370 Seventh Avenue, Suite 1200, New York, NY 10001
www.guilford.com

Printed in the United States of America

This book is printed on acid-free paper.

Last digit is print number: 9   8   7   6   5   4   3   2   1

The authors have checked with sources believed to be reliable in their efforts to provide
information that is complete and generally in accord with the standards of practice that are
accepted at the time of publication. However, in view of the possibility of human error or
changes in behavioral, mental health, or medical sciences, neither the authors, nor the editors
and publisher, nor any other party who has been involved in the preparation or publication
of this work warrants that the information contained herein is in every respect accurate or
complete, and they are not responsible for any errors or omissions or the results obtained from
the use of such information. Readers are encouraged to confirm the information contained in
this book with other sources.

Library of Congress Cataloging-in-Publication Data

Names: Holmes, Emily A., author.
Title: Imagery-based cognitive therapy for bipolar disorder and mood instability /
    Emily A. Holmes [and four others] ; foreword by Gillian Butler.
Description: New York : The Guilford Press, 2019. | Includes bibliographical references
    and index.
Identifiers: LCCN 2019005495 | ISBN 9781462539055 (paperback)
Subjects: LCSH: Manic–depressive illness—Treatment. | Cognitive therapy. | BISAC:
    PSYCHOLOGY / Psychopathology / Bipolar Disorder. | MEDICAL / Psychiatry / General. |
    SOCIAL SCIENCE / Social Work.
Classification: LCC RC516 .H65 2019 | DDC 616.89/5—dc23
LC record available at *https://lccn.loc.gov/2019005495*

IN MEMORY OF ANN HACKMANN

Like an explorer, you helped us to find
the haunting images within our minds.

Like a magician, you helped to change their nature,
elegantly conjuring ways to dispel them.

You shared ways to find calming images
and ways to find meaning.

You set up signposts along a road
including fun and occasional chaos—
the best road to be on.

About the Authors

Emily A. Holmes, DClinPsy, PhD, is Professor of Psychology in the Department of Psychology at Uppsala University in Uppsala, Sweden, and in the Department of Clinical Neuroscience at the Karolinska Institutet, Stockholm, Sweden. She is Visiting Professor of Clinical Psychology at the University of Oxford, United Kingdom. Her research and publications focus on mental imagery and emotion across psychological disorders. She is a clinical psychologist with a PhD in cognitive neuroscience. Dr. Holmes is an associate editor of *Behaviour Research and Therapy* and serves on the Board of Trustees of the international mental health research charity MQ: Transforming Mental Health. She is a recipient of the May Davidson Award from the British Psychological Society, the Comenius Early Career Award from the European Federation of Psychologists' Associations, and the Award for Distinguished Early Career Scientific Contribution to Psychology from the American Psychological Association, among other honors. She is a member of the Royal Swedish Academy of Sciences.

Susie A. Hales, DClinPsy, is Research Tutor and Clinical Psychologist at the Oxford Institute of Clinical Psychology Training, University of Oxford, and Oxford Health NHS Foundation Trust, United Kingdom. Her research focuses on mental imagery processes and treatment innovation for mood disorders. Dr. Hales has published papers on psychological aspects of bipolar disorder and suicidality, and on novel ways of delivering cognitive therapy. She is active in the supervision and training of mental health professionals in a range of research and clinical competencies, with a particular emphasis on the provision of imagery-focused cognitive therapy training workshops.

Kerry Young, DipClinPsy, is Consultant Clinical Psychologist and Clinical Lead of the Woodfield Trauma Service in London, United Kingdom. She is also Honorary Lecturer in Clinical Psychology at University College London and a clinician at the Oxford Rose Clinic.

Dr. Young is an expert in mental imagery techniques, particularly imagery rescripting and its use with clients who have experienced complex trauma. She has published in the area of trauma and mental imagery.

Martina Di Simplicio, MD, PhD, is Clinical Senior Lecturer in Psychiatry at the Centre for Psychiatry, Imperial College London, United Kingdom, and Honorary Consultant Psychiatrist in the West London NHS Trust. Her research focuses on understanding the cognitive mechanisms that underlie psychopathology and that drive successful treatment of mental disorders. Dr. Di Simplicio investigates the role of mental imagery in regulating emotions, with the aim of developing innovative digital interventions for young people who experience mood instability and self-harm. She has published on emotion processing, neuroimaging, psychopharmacology, and mental imagery.

Foreword

This is an unusually interesting and useful book. It introduces clinicians and their clients to a new set of techniques that are likely to make a big difference in the treatment of bipolar disorder (BD)—a problem that can bring with it a notoriously intractable set of difficulties. At the same time, it demonstrates an approach to the development of new ways of using cognitive-behavioral therapy (CBT) that may well have much wider application.

It is well known that CBT is based on clearly expressed principles that guide its application, and are linked to specific tools and techniques. These characteristics certainly contributed to its original success, and they can still make it seem straightforward (even easy) to apply. Protocols have been created for specific problems, and practitioners from a variety of backgrounds can be trained relatively quickly to apply them. All these characteristics have made CBT more widely accessible. However, they have also given rise to reservations about its wider value. One of these is that it is a relatively superficial method, and not appropriate for people with long-standing and complex problems.

Not so. CBT is versatile, and its more sophisticated applications, which combine principles-based work with a highly individualized approach, now help many people who suffer from chronic and complex problems. And here is another new development, this time conceptualized in an original way.

In this book, the authors focus not on another diagnostic category as a whole but on one of its aspects—and on one that has not, until recently, been seen as definitional. Imagery has been shown to be an "emotional amplifier"; so, it is suggested, the experience of images plays an important part in the maintenance of BD, because it triggers extreme fluctuations in mood together with understandable but unhelpful actions. The focus here is on working only with images, applying a clearly specified and focused set of techniques in what is described as the Mood Action Psychology Program (MAPP). MAPP involves "remapping" both the processes involved and our understanding of how images (not only visual ones) precipitate these extreme fluctuations in affect and behavior. The ability to recognize and understand these processes is informed by neuropsychological and imagery research, and the evidence presented suggests that the methods used here greatly increase the potential for controlling mood fluctuations, or "blips." The language used throughout this book is both accessible and destigmatizing.

The methods used in MAPP are both general and specific. The general ones include stylistic elements of CBT, with a special emphasis on the value of curiosity. Curiosity reflects interest in the experiences and point of view of another person, balanced with an admission that there is much we cannot know about others unless they tell us. It reflects a willingness to explore, to search for key meanings, and to work to devise alternative ways of seeing things—using imagery work rather than verbal challenges. The choice of possible specific methods is thus dependent upon both clients' and therapists' using their curiosity, and the style of CBT is admirably suited to this task.

Specific methods are drawn largely from imagery research, and the net has been cast wide so as to include, among other things, metacognitive techniques, imagery rescripting, imagery-competing tasks, and positive imagery work. Many well-known methods are drawn together here into a new "toolbox," with the overall aim of changing how the image makes the client *feel* and/or how the client *reacts to it.* The guiding principles underlying the application of MAPP tell us that what is happening within a mental image is interesting, but that how it makes the client *feel or act* is where we need to direct our attention as therapists. The many illustrative case examples and verbatim comments from clients serve to underline that when this aim is achieved, the occurrence of disturbing images is less destabilizing. Another most valuable contribution—one that helps therapists to target their chosen interventions with precision, and to select others if necessary—is the use of "microformulation." Again, microformulation is based on principles derived from fundamental research, and its purpose is to work out how the capture of attention by an image, in a particular case, plays a role in maintenance. This is the tool that brings the general and the particular together.

So the new method made available to us in this book, although it focuses on imagery, is at heart a cognitive method. Having understood the precise effect of a cognitive event (an image) on mood and action, a therapist and client, working collaboratively, can search for a precise, matching, and helpful antidote. A combination of rigor and flexibility is required, and as clinicians and researchers, the authors of this book demonstrate their clarity and creativity throughout. The end result is that complex ideas are made accessible. Doing so requires general and specific skills and sensitivity—the application of art as well as science.

This sophisticated use of CBT has potential for alleviating other problems as well as BD, if and when clients report repeated and disturbing images that are linked to their mood and their actions. This applies regardless of diagnosis, or indeed in the context of comorbidity; more specifically, it could be helpful following traumatic experiences and in some manifestations of social anxiety. In theory, whenever imagery contributes to maintenance, the application of the principles and the methods used in MAPP could make a difference.

GILLIAN BUTLER, PhD
Oxford, United Kingdom

Preface

This manual offers something new: a detailed, step-by-step guide to working with mental imagery. All four of us have an abiding curiosity about mental imagery in our clinical work. We have been curious about the way imagery has a powerful impact on our emotions, whether we are working with people after trauma (e.g., those experiencing the so-called intrusive images characteristic of posttraumatic stress disorder, or PTSD) or with clients who have a wide range of other mental health conditions. We have noticed that *negative* imagery can cause profound distress. And we have noticed that harnessing more *positive* imagery can be a rapid way to bring relief and to move forward.

Working with people with bipolar disorder (BD) over the previous few years, we were struck by the prominence of vivid mental images in their presentation. We already knew that thinking in images has a more powerful effect on emotion than does thinking in words. In addition, we discovered that people with BD considered their mental images to be more compelling than did those with unipolar depression. Putting these two findings together, we began to wonder whether emotional mental images might be acting as an "emotional amplifier" in BD, and thus contributing to mood instability (Holmes, Geddes, Colom, & Goodwin, 2008). If this were the case, then an intervention targeting mental imagery might help to improve mood stability in BD. We devised a 10-session imagery-based assessment and intervention to do just that; we called it the Mood Action Psychology Program (MAPP).

This book is an expanded version of the therapy manual we used in the original MAPP case series. It will be most useful to those who are already familiar with cognitive-behavioral therapy (CBT), although we do not think that readers must be members of a particular mental health profession to benefit from it. Moreover, we do not think that clinicians need to work with BD to use this manual. As we have stated above, our interest in imagery runs across all mental health conditions; in other words, it is *transdiagnostic*. We believe that this manual will be of great use to people working with mental images in *any* area of mental health. The techniques we describe have been tried and developed in treatments for other conditions, such as PTSD, social anxiety disorder/social phobia, agoraphobia, health anxiety, obsessive–compulsive disorder, depression, chronic pain, substance misuse, psychosis, and so forth. Indeed, all four of us have used the techniques regularly for clients with a range of different clinical conditions.

In any clinical case formulation, the first line of treatment approach should always be in accord with the existing evidence. We tend to turn to the use of imagery techniques with people who may not fit within a standard "evidence-based box." This might be due to comorbidity, to complexity, or to the client's and therapist's choice of treatment target, and so imagery may augment what otherwise can be offered. Since we see mental imagery as a causal mechanism in emotion and behavior generally, then adding an imagery-based approach to therapy seeks not to replace but to help *improve* our repertoire of treatment options (Holmes et al., 2018).

As already mentioned, this manual is a step-by-step guide, describing in practical detail how to work with mental images. We have always enjoyed attending training in which the trainer tells us exactly how to do things. Thus each technique in this manual is described in a series of easy steps. The Appendices are a series of reproducible handouts, and we provide agendas for each session. We have also written comprehensive scripts, suggesting words that therapists can use to introduce and undertake the techniques. We have included lots of troubleshooting tips based on our combined clinical experience, as well as many worked-through case examples and excerpts from clinical sessions. This book and the thinking behind the techniques can be shared directly with clients, who in our experience may enjoy this as part of transparent and collaborative working. We hope that by the time you, our readers, have finished this manual, you will feel confident about how to assess and intervene with mental imagery with any client, and will also be enthusiastic about the potential power and simplicity of working with mental imagery.

COVER PICTURE CREDIT AND EXPLANATION

The painting on the front cover is by Camille Corot. It is entitled *Italian Landscape* and depicts a calm countryside scene. In the imagery-based cognitive therapy approach we devised, clients often choose postcards as a visual *aide-mémoire* for important pieces of learning. This Corot painting reminded us of a postcard one client selected to represent a newfound sense of harmony and balance in relation to living with bipolar disorder. The postcard helped her remember that "while the weather may change, the earth underneath will always endure." This Corot image seems a fitting encapsulation of this sentiment.

A NOTE ABOUT THE WORD "APPRAISAL"

In this book, "appraisal" simply means the *meaning/verbal thoughts* that the person is having in the image, for example, "I am going to die." It is these verbal thoughts that generate each of the emotions in the image, for example, "fear."

Acknowledgments

There are many people we would like to acknowledge and thank for their contributions to this book:

- The MAPP team, including Heather Mitchell, Simon Blackwell, Lalitha Iyadurai, Ella James, Ian Clark, Helen Close, Anna Bevan, Rachel Manser, Beata Godlewska, Sophie Wallace Hadrill, Aisha Malik, Craig Steel, Fritz Renner, Alex Lau Zhu, Julie Ji, Peter Watson, and Mike Bonsall, and for CBT consultancy Chris Fairburn.
- Our colleagues in the Department of Psychiatry at the University of Oxford and in the Oxford Health National Health Service (NHS) Foundation Trust, particularly Guy Goodwin (see the Afterword) and John Geddes, as well as Mary-Jane Attenborrow, Andrea Cipriani, Digby Quested, and Val Paulley.
- Our colleagues in Cambridgeshire and Peterborough NHS Foundation Trust (CPFT) in Cambridge, including Rajini Ramana, Fiona Mackie, Nikolett Kabacs, Nimalee Kanakkahewa, Neil Hunt, and Leonora Brosan.
- Gitta Jacob for her consultancy on chair work.
- People who have kindly commented on drafts of this manual: Cid Dixon, Phil Lurie, Fran Brady, Sam Akbar, Adele Stevens, Millay Vann, Zoe Chessell, and Antonella Riccardi.
- Clinical psychologists who provided discussion and inspiration, including Ann Hackmann, Arnoud Arntz, Gillian Butler, Helen Kennerley, Melanie Fennel, Craig Steel, Deborah Lee, Khadj Rouf, David Kavanagh, Andri Steinþór Björnsson, Pete McEvoy, James Bennett-Levy, and Irene Oestrich.
- Other researchers in psychological science who have worked with our team exploring imagery, including Chantal Berna, Stephanie Burnett Heyes, Muriel Hagenaars, Antje Horsch, Annabel Ivins, Marie Kanstrup, Henrik Kessler, Olivia Kukacka, Tamara Lang, Klara Lauri, Susie Murphy, Sabine Nelis, Roger Ng, Arnaud Pictet, Victoria Pile, Kate Porcheret, Christien Slofstra, Clare Rathbone, Hannah Stratford, Renee Visser, Alisha Williams, and Marcella Woud.
- Jim Nageotte at The Guilford Press for immensely helpful and encouraging editing.

- Particular and huge thanks to Ella James for invaluable help with the manuscript.
- The Wellcome Trust for Clinical Fellowship No. WT088217 to Emily A. Holmes: *A Psychological Approach to Understanding and Treating Bipolar Disorder: Investigating New Cognitive Mechanisms.*
- Our families, including Nuala and David; Christina and Bernard; Dagmar and Oscar; Linda and Tony; Frankie, Joss, Astrid, Evie, and Josie; and Craig, Alan, Phil, and Cormac.
- And especially all our clients in MAPP, for together helping us to shape what we did.

Contents

PART I
Introduction

CHAPTER 1

Introduction to Bipolar Disorder

Bipolar disorder (BD) is characterized by recurring episodes of depression and mania or hypomania. Although most people with BD experience both extremes of mood, the fifth edition of the *Diagnostic and Statistical Manual of Mental Disorders* (DSM-5; American Psychiatric Association, 2013) requires only the presence of a single episode of mania to meet diagnostic criteria for BD Type I. There are different subtypes of BD, and these tend to be categorized according to the duration and intensity of the manic or hypomanic symptoms. Hence, in this chapter we first explain what constitutes a manic episode. Next, we discuss the different subtypes of BD in more detail and describe how depressive episodes fit within the diagnostic framework.

MANIA: THE DEFINING DIAGNOSTIC FEATURE OF BD

"Mania" can be defined as a period of abnormally high mood. In a manic episode, individuals with BD experience an excessive sense of elation, excitement, or irritable mood, in conjunction with abnormally high energy levels or hyperactivity. They tend to demonstrate an increase in goal-directed activities that can escalate from being very productive (e.g., finishing a number of projects at work) to a state of constantly jumping between tasks. These two core features (elated/irritable mood and hyperactivity) are accompanied by a variety of other symptoms, including a subjective sense that one's thoughts are racing; an unstoppable flow of ideas; feelings of overoptimism; and inflated self-esteem and grandiosity (a sense of superiority).

The high energy levels present in a manic episode are combined with a reduced need for sleep or even insomnia. Individuals often report sleeping little (e.g., fewer than 4 hours per night) without feeling tired. Other symptoms more likely to be noticed by others are distractibility, restlessness, and an accelerated speech rate, such that it can be difficult to interrupt a person in a conversation.

During a manic episode, an individual can appear more extroverted than usual or even disinhibited (e.g., being rude or lewd in a social situation). He or she may also engage in pleasurable but risky activities, such as overspending, speeding, unwise promiscuity, or excessive drinking or drug taking. This can lead the person to damage close relationships, come into contact with the police or medical services, or incur significant debt. In addition, during an episode of mania individuals may experience psychotic symptoms, such as hallucinations or delusions, typically with a grandiose or paranoid content.

MANIA, HYPOMANIA, AND THE DIFFERENCE BETWEEN BD TYPES I AND II

The presence of full-blown mania means that an individual meets the DSM-5 criteria for BD Type I (American Psychiatric Association, 2013). BD Type II is the diagnosis used in cases where individuals have experienced one or more hypomanic episodes, as well as at least one depressive episode. "Hypomania" refers to symptoms (lasting for at least 4 consecutive days) of abnormally high mood that are milder than the symptoms of full-blown mania; individuals' usual mood and behavior may be altered, but they are still able to function in their everyday lives.

In reality, it is rare for individuals to experience mania only. Most individuals with BD also experience episodes of depression that alternate with episodes of mania or hypomania (in BD Type I) or of hypomania only (BD Type II). In fact, individuals with either type of BD tend to spend about three times longer in depressed than in manic or hypomanic mood states (Kupka et al., 2007).

DEPRESSIVE EPISODES

Depressive episodes are characterized by depressed (low) mood, a lack of motivation, and an inability to enjoy or gain pleasure from usually enjoyed activities ("anhedonia"). Together with these core features, individuals with depression can experience: low energy levels; a disturbed pattern of sleep and appetite; difficulty making decisions; trouble concentrating; and memory problems. Individuals may appear to speak or move slowly, or alternatively may be restless and agitated. Moreover, a typical pattern of negative thinking is present, including feelings of guilt, hopelessness, and helplessness about the self, the world, and the future. Suicidal thinking and/or behavior may occur in more severe episodes of depression.

In comparison with unipolar depression, it has been suggested that in bipolar depression there may be an increased incidence of psychosis; more diurnal mood variation (typically, feeling worse in the morning but better as the day progresses); increased hypersomnia (excessive sleepiness); and a larger overall number of depressive episodes over time, but tending to have a shorter duration (Forty et al., 2008).

"MIXED FEATURES" IN BD

Some individuals with BD also experience both manic and depressive symptoms concurrently in the same episode, or they may have rapid (even hourly) swings between mania and depression. These experiences are known as "mixed features." For example, an individual may appear restless and agitated, with accelerated thoughts, speech, and actions, but may still experience depressive cognitions and low mood.

OTHER TYPES OF BD

Besides the more common BD Types I and II, other types of BD as defined by DSM-5 include cyclothymic disorder; substance-induced (e.g., by stimulants) or medication-induced (e.g., by corticosteroids) BD; BD due to another medical condition (e.g., hyperthyroidism); and other specified or unspecified bipolar and related disorder.

Cyclothymic disorder is a chronic condition of fluctuating mood disturbance involving numerous periods of hypomanic symptoms and numerous periods of depressive symptoms over a period of at least 2 years. However, in this subtype neither the hypomanic nor the depressive symptoms are severe or pervasive enough to meet full criteria for a hypomanic or depressive episode.

The diagnosis of "other specified bipolar and related disorder" is applied when the symptoms of mood disturbance are characteristic of one of the above-described types of BD, but *do not* meet the full criteria for any of these disorders. Examples include hypomanic episodes of fewer than 4 days or with insufficient symptoms. All of these manifestations also fall into the category of "bipolar spectrum conditions" (Geddes & Miklowitz, 2013). The label "unspecified bipolar and related disorder" is used when bipolar symptoms are present but there is not enough information to make a more specific diagnosis, or when a clinician chooses not to give the reasons for not making a more specific diagnosis.

A NOTE ON BD AND DSM-5

The symptoms and features of BD vary hugely from individual to individual (Nandi, Beard, & Galea, 2009). The recently introduced DSM-5 system emphasizes a dimensional approach to diagnosis (American Psychiatric Association, 2013), in which the different types of BD are no longer considered as separate disorders but as related conditions on a continuum of behaviors, with some conditions reflecting mild symptoms (e.g., cyclothymia) and others much more severe symptoms (e.g., BD Type I). DSM-5 has also included so-called "specifiers" that better account for the heterogeneous clinical presentations of BD. Clinicians can specify characteristics that may be prominent for some individuals and that can influence clinical management, such as a rapid-cycling course, postpartum onset, psychotic symptoms, or anxiety. This gives clinicians the potential to individualize treatment approaches further.

EPIDEMIOLOGY

The prevalence of BD is estimated at 1–4% of the general population (Kroon et al., 2013), equally distributed between genders. The peak age at onset of BD spans adolescence and early adulthood (15–24 years) (Merikangas et al., 2011), and BD is usually a lifelong disorder, with 50–60% of people relapsing within 1 year of recovery from an episode (Kessing, Hansen, & Andersen, 2004).

SUICIDALITY AND QUALITY OF LIFE IN BD

The impact of BD can vary widely. One of the most sobering statistics related to BD concerns suicidality. Individuals with BD have the highest suicide rate of all the psychiatric disorders (Hawton, Sutton, Haw, Sinclair, & Harriss, 2005), with 10–20% of people diagnosed with BD taking their own lives, and nearly one-third admitting to at least one suicide attempt (Müller-Oerlinghausen, Berghöfer, & Bauer, 2002). Rates of self-harm are also high, with about 10–14% of this population presenting at hospitals after a self-inflicted injury (Webb, Lichtenstein, Larsson, Geddes, & Fazel, 2014).

Research suggests that individuals with BD have a lower quality of life in all domains, compared to healthy individuals of the same age (Rademacher, DelBello, Adler, Stanford, & Strakowski, 2007). It has also been suggested that of all the mental disorders, BD is associated with the greatest reduction in potential personal and professional achievement, when pre- to postillness adjustment and functioning are compared (Scott, 2011). This impact on functioning is likely to be linked with the chronic mood instability that persists even when an individual has recovered from an episode of mania/hypomania or depression (Henry et al., 2008; Hirschfeld et al., 2007). Until recently, the traditional view has been that people with BD experience periods of "euthymia" (normal, nondepressed, stable mood) between mood episodes. However, studies carried out in the last few years have shown that the majority of individuals with BD experience mood fluctuations at subsyndromal levels for most of their lives (Birmaher et al., 2014; Judd et al., 2002), with these fluctuations being linked to a worse prognosis and overall level of functioning (Bopp, Miklowitz, Goodwin, Rendell, & Geddes, 2010; Strejilevich et al., 2013).

Another important factor that has a large impact on the lives of individuals with BD is the frequency of comorbid disorders: One large-scale survey showed that out of 9,000 people with a diagnosis of BD, 92% had at least one comorbidity (Merikangas et al., 2007). The most common comorbid diagnoses are substance misuse (rated at about 50% lifetime comorbidity; Cassidy, Ahearn, & Carroll, 2001) and anxiety. In the next section, we discuss the significance of anxiety disorder comorbidity, and examine how it intersects with another significant feature of BD: the presence of emotional mental imagery.

BIPOLAR ANXIETY: A TRACTABLE TARGET FOR PSYCHOLOGICAL INTERVENTION

Lifetime rates of anxiety comorbidity in BD are extremely high: In the U.S. National Comorbidity Survey Replication, as many as 90% of individuals with BD Type I reported having had an anxiety disorder at some time (Freeman, Freeman, & McElroy, 2002; Merikangas et al., 2007). The most recent meta-analysis of 40 studies, including 14,914 individuals from North America, Europe, Australia, South America, and Asia, suggested a lifetime prevalence of anxiety disorders in BD of about 45% (Pavlova, Perlis, Alda, & Uher, 2015).

How does the presence of anxiety add to the impact of BD? We know that the presence of anxiety in BD is a major contributory factor to poor functioning (Kroon et al., 2013) and is closely linked to a worse prognosis (Otto et al., 2006). Anxiety comorbidity is also associated with a higher risk (and longer duration) of depressive relapses, with less time spent in euthymic mood between episodes, and higher rates of hospitalization and use of psychotropic medication (Fagiolini et al., 2007). It is also linked with increased rapid cycling of mood states and higher suicidal risk (Simon et al., 2007). Intriguingly, evidence also suggests that the presence of anxiety in young people at the prodromal stages of bipolar spectrum disorder predicts a longitudinal course toward the full-blown disorder (Skjelstad, Malt, & Holte, 2010). Therefore, it would seem clear that addressing anxiety symptoms in treatment may be critical to attaining full recovery.

Recently published treatment guidelines from the British Association of Psychopharmacology (BAP) (Goodwin et al., 2016) have highlighted the need for future research that will enable us to better understand and treat anxiety comorbidity within the BD population. Specifically, there is a need to understand whether there are bipolar-specific features of anxiety that go beyond simple comorbidity with other anxiety disorders. Because both anxiety symptoms and subsyndromal mood instability persist during periods of normal mood, and because we know that they have such a profound impact on functioning and prognosis, understanding the relationship between these two phenomena could be crucial to improving the well-being of individuals with BD.

THE IMPACT OF EMOTIONAL MENTAL IMAGERY

The increased prevalence of anxiety in BD may be linked to the high levels of "emotional mental imagery" experienced by this population. Our research group has investigated many aspects of this phenomenon in BD, and we have proposed that vivid intrusive mental imagery may act as an "emotional amplifier" that may drive both anxiety and the escalation of mood states in BD (Holmes, Geddes, Colom, & Goodwin, 2008). For example, many people with BD experience anxiety-provoking vivid, negative, future-related mental imagery. These negative mental images may amplify the expectation of future threat, causing anxiety or low mood, and thereby contributing to mood instability (Holmes et al., 2011). Similarly, "flashforward" images of fantasy suicidal acts have been reported as more compelling in persons with BD than in individuals with unipolar depression (Hales, Deeprose, Goodwin, & Holmes, 2011). Conversely, vivid positive mental imagery is also rated as more exciting in BD than in unipolar depression and is associated with greater levels of behavioral activation (Ivins, Di Simplicio, Close, Goodwin, & Holmes, 2014). Thus we can see how, for people with BD, experiencing more intrusive and compelling mental images may act as a driver for mood instability.

Greater susceptibility to experiencing intrusive mental imagery (Malik, Goodwin, Hoppitt, & Holmes, 2014; Ng, Burnett Heyes, McManus, Kennerley, & Holmes, 2016; Ng, Di Simplicio, McManus, Kennerley, & Holmes, 2016), and a greater tendency for vivid mental imagery to escalate mood (O'Donnell, Di Simplicio, Brown, Holmes, & Burnett Heyes, 2018), have also been described in healthy samples with a high vulnerability to BD (i.e., persons scoring highly on trait measures of BD). These findings suggest that characteristics of mental imagery may be relevant for the whole BD spectrum, not just those people meeting full criteria for a BD diagnosis. Moreover, in a recent experimental study, mental imagery characteristics (such as the vividness of negative future imagery and the impact of intrusive images) appeared to be associated with anxiety severity and mood variability across different diagnoses (Di Simplicio et al., 2016). This suggests that mental imagery could be a specific target for intervention in many diagnoses.

In BD, where anxiety and mood instability symptoms are frequently intertwined with vivid and compelling mental images, it would seem sensible to explore the potential of taking these experimental findings out of the laboratory and into the clinical field. The members of our group have done this, and we have shown in a clinical case series that an imagery-focused intervention, known as the Mood Action Psychology Program (MAPP), is able to reduce anxiety and mood instability in BD (Holmes, Bonsall, et al., 2016). More information about the development and implementation of this intervention can be found in Chapter 2 and beyond.

CURRENT TREATMENT APPROACHES TO BD

Pharmacological approaches to treating BD have predominated for many years, but more recently, psychological treatments have been developed, tested, and shown to be effective. We briefly review the main drug treatments for BD before describing more recent psychological treatments.

Pharmacological Approaches

All international guidelines for the treatment of BD recommend that BD be predominantly managed with medication such as mood stabilizers (American Psychiatric Association, 2002; Yatham et al., 2013; National Institute for Health and Care Excellence [NICE], 2014). Frequently prescribed medications include lithium, valproate, olanzapine, risperidone, quetiapine, and lamotrigine. However, these medications have varying degrees of success for the treatment of acute episodes and the prevention of relapses. For further information, see the BAP treatment guidelines for BD (Goodwin et al., 2016) and the International College of Neuro-Psychopharmacology (CINP) treatment guidelines for BD in adults (Fountoulakis et al., 2017).

While pharmacotherapy remains the mainstay of treatment for BD, frequent relapses remain common, with one study reporting that 37% of individuals with BD had a recurrence of depression or mania within 1 year and 60% within 2 years (Perlis et al., 2006). Furthermore, individuals with BD tend to experience residual depressive symptoms for one-third of their lives (Judd et al., 2002), with a corresponding impact on functioning and quality of life. Treating and preventing relapses of depression remain major treatment challenges, with only a handful of medications (lamotrigine, lithium, and quetiapine) showing convincing effects in this respect (Yatham et al., 2013; Goodwin et al., 2016). Moreover, the use of antidepressants to target depression in BD remains controversial, as these drugs may contribute to shifting individuals from a depressed state into mania; this phenomenon is often referred to as a "manic switch" (Baldessarini et al., 2013; Pacchiarotti et al., 2013).

The Enhanced Care Approach

Alongside medication, another mainstay of BD management is a model of "enhanced care," whereby clinicians aim to establish a good therapeutic alliance with clients and to involve caregivers or significant others in their care. Both strategies aim to ensure that individuals with BD engage in long-term monitoring of their mood and (often) a long-term medication regimen. This approach was also endorsed in the BAP treatment guidelines (Goodwin et al., 2016) as follows: "Partners, families and carers can contribute significantly to the assessment process, the management of acute episodes, the promotion of long-term recovery and the prevention of relapse."

Enhanced care also involves clinicians' providing psychoeducation to both clients and caregivers about important factors affecting the course of BD. The topics covered tend to include the impact of stressors on mood, ways to manage sleep disturbance, the early signs of relapse, and the importance of regular activity patterns (NICE, 2014). While structured manualized protocols of group psychoeducation have been proven effective at reducing depressive relapses (Colom et al., 2009), it is also recommended that psychoeducation become part of good clinical practice for all people diagnosed with BD (Goodwin et al., 2016; NICE, 2014).

Psychological Approaches

The American Psychiatric Association (2002) guidelines highlight that specific forms of psychotherapy are critical components of the treatment plan for many patients with BD, alongside medication. In particular, these guidelines advocate psychological treatments aimed at reducing distress, improving the patient's functioning between episodes and decreasing the likelihood of relapse. However, they conclude that the choice of psychological intervention will vary, depending on clinicians' expertise and patients' preferences. Similarly, in the United Kingdom, NICE (2014) recommends specific psychological treatments for people with BD, either to (1) prevent relapse or (2) treat persisting symptoms between episodes of mania or bipolar depression. In these cases, the advice is to "offer a structured psychological intervention (individual, group or family), which has been designed for bipolar disorder and has a published evidence-based manual describing how it should be delivered."

The main psychological treatment approaches tested in clinical trials so far have been family therapy interventions, interpersonal and social rhythms therapy (IPSRT), and cognitive-behavioral therapy (CBT). However, the evidence for the effectiveness of various psychological interventions for BD is mixed and sometimes contested (Jauhar, McKenna, & Laws, 2016). Recent attempts at comparing different interventions have also highlighted that the evidence is too scarce and heterogeneous for reliable conclusions to be drawn (Chatterton et al., 2017; Miklowitz, Cipriani, & Goodwin, 2017).

A possible reason for this lack of efficacy is that many treatments and models used for BD have been adjusted from those provided for depression and psychosis, rather than developed specifically for BD and its unique features and challenges. This is particularly true for CBT protocols.

Family therapy protocols are based on the use of psychoeducation and some CBT principles for people with BD and their caregivers. There is an additional focus on improving communication within the family and on problem-solving skills. Family therapy (when compared with usual care) has been found to be effective in reducing depressive relapses and improving social functioning over a 30-month follow-up (Miklowitz, Goodwin, Bauer, & Geddes, 2008). However, a family-based approach may not be suited to all individuals, nor is it necessarily superior to good-quality pharmacological care (Miklowitz et al., 2014).

IPSRT for acute depressive episodes also includes psychoeducation but has an additional emphasis on modifying interpersonal factors, promoting good sleep schedules, and encouraging regular daily activities. It has been shown to reduce relapse over a 2-year follow-up (Frank et al., 2005). However, a recent systematic review concluded that it was not clear whether IPSRT was of greater benefit than an intensive supportive care intervention of similar duration (Crowe, Beaglehole, & Inder, 2016).

A large randomized controlled trial reported that CBT for BD was effective in reducing depressive relapses and enhancing social functioning in clients over a 24-month follow-up period (Lam, Hayward, Watkins, Wright, & Sham, 2005). However, subsequent trials disappointingly failed to replicate the results (Scott et al., 2006; Zaretsky, Lancee, Miller, Harris, & Parikh, 2008). Still, there are indications that the CBT approach may yet be useful for individuals with a more recent onset and fewer mood episodes (Scott et al., 2006). More recent studies have also highlighted the importance of focusing on more personalized recovery goals (Jones et al., 2015), in addition to traditional outcomes such as mood relapse.

In summary, there is some limited evidence to suggest that psychological therapies in their current form benefit individuals with BD in preventing relapses. The key ingredients of all psychotherapies so far found useful for BD are summarized in the BAP guidelines as follows (after Miklowitz et al., 2008):

1. Monitor moods and early warning signs.
2. Recognize and manage stress triggers and interpersonal conflicts.
3. Develop relapse prevention plans.
4. Stabilize sleep–wake rhythms and daily routines.
5. Encourage medication adherence.
6. Reduce self-stigmatization.
7. Reduce alcohol or drug use (including caffeine use in sensitive individuals).

A NOTE ON THE TREATMENT OF ANXIETY IN THE CONTEXT OF BD

As we have discussed, anxiety comorbidity may be a significant characteristic of BD. International guidelines disagree on the preferred treatment approach for anxiety comorbidity, with some indicating pharmacological approaches alongside mindfulness-based interventions (Fountoulakis et al., 2017), and others focusing more on psychological therapies (Yatham et al., 2013). Pharmacological approaches to treating anxiety comorbidity are limited by the need for extreme caution in using antidepressants (which are often prescribed as antianxiety agents), due to the risk of "manic switch." Therefore, psychological interventions may be particularly helpful in this regard.

The current NICE (2014) guidelines for BD treatment recommend that when anxiety is present, the psychological intervention indicated for the specific comorbid anxiety disorder identified (e.g., social anxiety disorder/social phobia) should be offered. Similarly, the American Psychiatric Association (2002) guidelines indicate that treatment for anxiety and for BD should proceed concurrently. A few studies have specifically looked at the efficacy of psychological interventions for anxiety within BD, with some indication of positive effects of CBT. Nevertheless, tailored approaches for anxiety in BD are lacking (Stratford, Blackwell, Di Simplicio, Cooper, & Holmes, 2014). Moreover, not all people with BD will meet full criteria for an anxiety disorder. This, together with the fact that BD is typically an exclusion criterion in the trials of psychological treatments for anxiety, suggests that the NICE recommendations at best "represent extrapolation" (Goodwin et al., 2016).

Nevertheless, clinical experience suggests that individuals with BD experience pervasive anxiety, which is distressing and has a significant impact on functioning, but which manifests as subclinical symptoms of multiple different anxiety diagnoses. Identifying the "correct" anxiety intervention protocol to apply can be problematic. Thus it may be more sensible to identify specific psychological treatment components that can reduce anxiety in BD. The BAP guidelines suggest that one such component might be strategies that are known to reduce the intensity of mental imagery. However, these guidelines conclude that further research and development are required (Goodwin et al., 2016).

CONCLUDING COMMENTS

In summary, despite a huge amount of research activity in the field of BD, the potential benefits of combining medication and psychotherapy need to be more closely examined. To quote the BAP guidelines, there is a "widely perceived need for closer integration between psychological and pharmacological interventions" (Goodwin et al., 2016). Furthermore, the treatment of anxiety within BD is currently a neglected target for intervention, but one that will likely prove particularly fruitful to pursue and evaluate, given the impact of anxiety on other facets of BD.

In this manual, we describe how our group developed MAPP, a psychological treatment for BD (to be used alongside any pharmacological intervention) that targets intrusive and emotional mental imagery. Our general goal has been to minimize the mood-destabilizing effects of intrusive imagery and equip clients with a potent tool that they can use now and in the future. In the next chapter, we delineate the science behind our understanding of mental imagery, its role in the etiology of psychopathology, and its use in treating psychological difficulties. The remainder of the book explains the various components of the treatment and illustrates its clinical implementation. Our aim is to provide the reader with background knowledge about mental imagery; a clear idea of MAPP's structure; guidance regarding how to assess and formulate mental images and then choose an intervention strategy; and, finally, direction on precisely how to undertake each of the strategies.

CHAPTER 2

Introduction to Mental Imagery and the Development of MAPP

In Chapter 1, we have described the main features of and contemporary treatments for BD. We have also proposed an imagery-based approach to treating BD, called MAPP. In this chapter, we explain why we believe that mental images may play an active role in the maintenance of BD, and why we think that working with these images may improve the effectiveness of psychotherapy. Then we describe the development and implementation of MAPP. We begin with a discussion of mental imagery and how it functions.

WHAT IS MENTAL IMAGERY?

Mental images form a significant part of how we think about the world and react to events around us. Kosslyn, Ganis, and Thompson (2001) have provided a useful definition:

> Mental imagery occurs when perceptual information is accessed from memory, giving rise to the experience of "seeing with the mind's eye," "hearing with the mind's ear" and so on. By contrast, perception occurs when information is directly registered from the senses. Mental images need not result simply in the recall of previously perceived objects or events; they can also be created by combining and modifying stored perceptual information in novel ways.

In other words, mental images are sensory events that occur inside someone's mind without a corresponding current stimulus in the outside world. They can be "rendered" in a single sense (sight, sound, taste, smell, or somatic sensation) or in more than one sense (e.g., a visual image of one's mother plus the sound of her voice, the smell of her perfume, or the touch of her hand). Mental images can be fleeting, or they may last for longer. They can also be static or moving, clear or blurred. They can be drawn from memories or may reflect novel or even impossible combinations of elements. Just as verbal thoughts can be, mental images can be retrieved deliberately or involuntarily, cued by an internal or external stimulus. Mental images can have positive, neutral, or negative content. Most of us may become aware of mental images and the extent to which they are present in our lives only when we start to pay attention to them.

How Does Mental Imagery Fit In with CBT?

From his first published works, Aaron T. Beck emphasized the importance of mental images in understanding psychological distress (Beck, 1970; Beck & Emery with Greenberg, 1985). He argued that images, memories, dreams, and nightmares often hold important information about people's appraisals of themselves, the world, and others. Rachman (1980, 2001) developed these ideas further in his work on "emotional processing." He argued that intrusive negative images and memories are often markers of a lack of emotional processing, and that a reduction in these phenomena should be expected after successful psychological interventions. Peter Lang (1977) pioneered the use of imagery techniques, seeing emotional mental images as simulations of reality. (For a review in tribute to Lang's work for the 50th anniversary of the Association for Behavioral and Cognitive Therapies, see Ji, Burnett Heyes, MacLeod, & Holmes, 2016.)

Awareness of the importance of mental imagery in CBT has increased in recent years. From clinical research, we discover that across many disorders, clients' intense emotional reactions or states are accompanied by vivid mental images. Mental imagery is well established as being a central component of posttraumatic stress disorder (PTSD) and intrusive memories of trauma (e.g., Ehlers & Clark, 2000), and has also been discovered in specific phobias (Pratt, Cooper, & Hackmann, 2004), obsessive–compulsive disorder (OCD) (de Silva, 1986), social anxiety disorder/social phobia (Wells & Clark, 1997), depression (Brewin, Watson, McCarthy, Hyman, & Dayson, 1998), bulimia nervosa (Somerville, Cooper, & Hackmann, 2007), health anxiety (Muse, McManus, Hackmann, & Williams, 2010), body dysmorphic disorder (BDD) (Osman, Cooper, Hackmann, & Veale, 2004), substance misuse (Kavanagh, Andrade, & May, 2005), schizophrenia (Morrison et al., 2002), and BD (Holmes, Geddes, et al., 2008). Readers wanting more information about the presence of mental imagery across disorders are referred to the opening chapters of the *Oxford Guide to Imagery in Cognitive Therapy* (Hackmann, Bennett-Levy, & Holmes, 2011; Holmes & Mathews, 2010).

While it is clear that emotional mental images are a crucial part of many psychological disorders, interventions that target mental images are not as widely known as those targeting verbal thoughts. In this chapter, we introduce the most commonly used techniques for working with mental imagery. Then, in the rest of the book, we describe in practical, step-by-step detail how we have applied many of these techniques with people suffering from BD.

COMMONLY USED TECHNIQUES FOR WORKING WITH MENTAL IMAGES

In order to help us organize our thoughts about imagery techniques, Holmes, Arntz, and Smucker (2007) suggest distinguishing between techniques that involve *directly* working with an image (generally either evoking or manipulating an image) and those that involve working *indirectly* with the image (e.g., metacognitive approaches). Furthermore, they suggest that these direct and indirect techniques can also be viewed in terms of whether they involve reducing negative imagery or promoting positive imagery (see Figure 2.1).

Direct Techniques

The direct techniques, as just mentioned, enable a therapist and client to focus on working with the images themselves. Here, we describe the key direct techniques commonly used in treatment.

Imaginal Exposure

Imaginal exposure involves deliberately evoking a troublesome image. Typically, the client is asked to bring to mind the image and recount in detail what he or she can see, hear, taste, smell, feel, and think, as follows:

> "I am going to ask you what you can see, hear, smell, taste, and feel in the image . . . all of the details. Also, about what happens in the image and when. This is because I want to be able to understand it well enough to see it myself, inside my own head. When

	Targeting NEGATIVE imagery	Enhancing POSITIVE imagery
Imagery-content-focused **Direct techniques**	Imaginal exposure	Scripting compassion-focused imagery
	Imagery rescripting of intrusive (image-based) memories	Building positive future-self images
	Imagery rescripting of fantasy images	
Imagery-property-focused **Indirect techniques**	Mindfulness-based cognitive therapy	
	Metacognitive image-based interventions	Imagery-based positive interpretation training
	Visuospatial imagery-competing tasks	

FIGURE 2.1. An illustration of the distinction between direct and indirect techniques, as well as between working to reduce negative images and working to promote positive images. Based on Holmes, Arntz, and Smucker (2007).

was the last time that you had that image? Now close your eyes and take yourself back to that moment: What were you doing? Where were you? Now can you get the image back in your head? Is it there? Now can you describe it to me in the first person and the present tense—for example, 'I can see X and I can hear Y'?"

Imaginal exposure can provide useful information for assessing intrusive images, and it has been a fundamental part of treatment for anxiety disorders since the beginnings of CBT (e.g., Foa & Rothbaum, 1998; Shapiro, 2001; Stampfl & Levis, 1967; Wolpe, 1958).

There is much debate about the mechanism(s) of change during imaginal exposure when it is used as a treatment for anxiety disorders. However, most clinicians and researchers would agree that during imaginal exposure, clients are able to reflect upon and possibly reappraise their negative mental images. Clients also learn that they can cope with holding those images in mind.

Restructuring Fantasy Images

Many people experience exaggerated or distorted mental images of anxiety-provoking situations, often called "fantasy images." For instance, clients who fear dogs may realize that whenever they see a dog, they experience a vivid image of it jumping up and biting them. Having identified and elaborated this fantasy image, a therapist could discuss with such a client how realistic it is, and help the client think about how to restructure/change the image. Alternatively, as in all areas of CBT, "behavioral experiments" can be used to test predictions contained in fantasy images. For example, clients who experience vivid mental images of themselves looking anxious in meetings at work may avoid meetings altogether or may become extremely anxious when one begins. The therapist can help such a client explore the image and then devise a behavioral experiment to test whether what the client sees in the image is true. This experiment might involve the client's videoing him- or herself in a meeting or asking others, "How do I look in meetings?" This information could then be used to correct or restructure the client's fantasy image.

Rescripting Image-Based Intrusive Memories

If imaginal exposure alone does not promote spontaneous reappraisal of negative images, then "rescripting" can be brought in to help the process along. Verbal rescripting involves introducing new verbal information into imaginal exposure. For example, in PTSD, the client may be asked to relive the traumatic event (e.g., a car crash) and then introduce updated verbal information at points of peak emotion (saying, "I survived," at the point in the account of the crash where the client had thought he or she was going to die) (Ehlers & Clark, 2000; Grey, Young, & Holmes, 2002). With imaginal rescripting, the updated information takes the form of an image rather than words (e.g., for the same car crash, an image of the client alive and well today).

Rescripting a troubling or negative image using another image is often employed when a verbal update/rescripting does not produce a strong enough change in affect. It can also be crucial when a change in somatic sensations is needed. For example, Jung and Steil

(2013) describe a powerful three-session intervention for adult survivors of childhood abuse who presented with persistent feelings of contamination alongside PTSD. The clients were encouraged to research using the internet/medical texts whether it was still possible for their bodies to contain the body fluids of their abusers. They all discovered that the cells in question had "turned over" hundreds or thousands of times since the abuse. Next, they were encouraged to generate and practice an image that represented this information about the renewal of their cells. Finally, they were asked to "bring on" the old feelings of contamination and then swap in the new, "clean" images.

Imaginal rescripting can also be useful to change what happens in an intrusive memory. For example, a therapist can help a client rescript memories of childhood abuse by getting the client to introduce (in imagination) adults to protect and comfort the child who has been abused, or to prevent the abuse (e.g., Arntz, Sofi, & van Breukelen, 2013; Layden, Newman, Freeman, & Byers Morse, 1993; Smucker, Dancu, Foa, & Niederee, 1995; Weertman & Arntz, 2007). Indeed, in the field of PTSD, exposure plus some form of verbal or imaginal rescripting tends to have some superior effects to exposure alone (e.g., Arntz, Tiesema, & Kindt, 2007; Ehlers et al., 2003).

Recent research has also shown the potential of extending rescripting of negative intrusive images to other disorders, such as depression (Wheatley et al., 2007) and social phobia (Wild, Hackmann, & Clark, 2007, 2008). Similarly, as already mentioned, using evidence gained during *in vivo* exposure, clients can successfully rescript fantasy/distorted images (e.g., of giant, aggressive snakes in snake phobias; Hunt & Fenton, 2007). A recent meta-analysis concluded that imagery rescripting is a promising intervention for a range of psychological complaints related to aversive memories, "with large effects obtained in a small number of sessions" (Morina, Lancee, & Arntz, 2017).

In Chapter 9, we explain rescripting techniques in detail.

Building Positive Imagery

In recent years, CBT therapists have sought to promote more positive, balanced imagery rather than focusing only on changing negative images. Evidence from neuroscience, sports psychology, and cognitive science points to the strong impact of positive images on emotions (e.g., Decety & Grèzes, 2006; Holmes, Mathews, Dalgleish, & Mackintosh, 2006; Holmes, Mathews, Mackintosh, & Dalgleish, 2008) and to the benefits of using imagery in goal setting and skills development (Cumming & Ramsey, 2008; Jones & Stuth, 1997; Renner et al., 2019).

Positive image generation can help in a number of quite different scenarios:

1. Rehearsing anxiety-provoking situations to increase confidence—for example, in the treatment of social phobia (Wild et al., 2007, 2008).
2. Rehearsing undertaking homework tasks to increase compliance in CBT (Beck, 2005)—for example, in depression when positive future is imagery lacking (Holmes, Lang, Moulds, & Steele, 2008).
3. "Fleshing out" goals for the future, to increase compliance with taking steps toward the goals—for example, in study skills research (Greitemeyer & Wurz, 2006; MacLeod, Coates, & Hetherton, 2008; Renner et al., 2019).

4. Compassionate Mind Training (Gilbert, 2009; Gilbert & Irons, 2005; Lee, 2005), which involves (among other things) generating an image to help a self-attacking client experience feelings of compassion and care. It can involve constructing a "perfect nurturer" (Lee, 2005) in imagination, which can be used regularly to guide the client toward self-compassion.
5. Constructing new, more helpful mental representations of oneself—for example, in Competitive Memory Training (COMET; Korrelboom, de Jong, Huijbrechts, & Daansen, 2009; Korrelboom, Marissen, & van Assendelft, 2011; Korrelboom, Van der Gaag, Hendriks, Huijbrechts, & Berretty, 2008; Korrelboom, van der Weele, Gjaltema, & Hoogstraten, 2009), which involves (among other techniques) using imagery, posture, and music to strengthen and make more vivid personal memories containing positive representations of oneself. These are then practiced regularly to increase the likelihood of their being accessed in preference to more negative memories.
6. Being used as a stand-alone technique to promote positive or safe feelings.

Chapter 7 contains information to clarify the neuroscience behind the apparent power of mental imagery in changing emotions. Chapter 10 has more details about how to generate and use positive imagery.

Indirect Techniques

The indirect techniques, as mentioned earlier, do not involve direct manipulation of the content of mental images. Rather, they involve understanding and working with the properties of these images. Here, we describe the key indirect techniques commonly used in treatment.

Metacognitive Techniques

Metacognitive techniques are a group of strategies aimed at lessening an image's impact on a client by changing how he or she relates to it. These techniques reinforce that the image is "just an image," not a physical reality, and that the client does not have to pay attention to the image and should direct attention elsewhere. In most cases, there is no real engagement with the content of the image. Metacognitive techniques fall into two main categories:

1. "Switching techniques," in which the client switches the focus of attention from internal images to the outside world—for example, focusing on the sight/texture/sound of objects in the outside.
2. "Image property techniques," in which the client changes the image in a way that reinforces its unreality—for example, imagining popping the image like a balloon, shrinking, changing its color or making it look comical.

Chapter 8 contains more information about using metacognitive techniques to work with mental imagery.

Imagery-Competing Tasks

One novel approach to treating or managing troublesome images is to disrupt or interfere with them using competing visuospatial tasks—tasks that have a significant visual and/or spatial component, such as playing a visual computer game or playing football. Competing tasks are often used when a client is troubled by a high volume of different images and needs an immediate coping strategy to help reduce the negative impact of images.

The use of competing visuospatial tasks to manage troublesome mental images has its roots in cognitive psychological research (e.g., Engelhard, van den Hout, Janssen, & van der Beek, 2010; Holmes, James, Coode-Bate, & Deeprose, 2009; Iyadurai et al., 2018; James et al., 2015; Kavanagh, Freese, Andrade, & May, 2001). In essence, these studies have found that if a client undertakes a concurrent visuospatial task while thinking about a troublesome visual image, both the vividness and emotionality of the image can be diminished. Researchers hypothesize that this effect occurs because the image and the visuospatial task compete for the limited visual processing space within the client's mind.

Chapter 11 gives details of how to use competing visuospatial tasks to manage troublesome images.

Positive Interpretation Training

The relatively new field of computerized "cognitive bias modification" (CBM; Koster, Fox, & MacLeod, 2009; MacLeod, Koster, & Fox, 2009) takes as its starting point the assumption that some psychological difficulties (e.g., depression) are associated with cognitive processing biases (e.g., "glass half empty" thinking). CBM paradigms involve using computers to train participants repeatedly to resolve ambiguous scenarios in a positive way, with the aim of reversing the bias. Researchers have found that the effect of CBM can be greater if participants imagine the positive outcomes rather than simply processing them verbally (Holmes et al., 2006). So far, there is only limited evidence that imagery-focused positive training can improve anhedonia (but not all depressive symptoms) in people with clinical depression (Blackwell & Holmes, 2010; Blackwell et al., 2015); however, further research is needed.

THE DEVELOPMENT OF MAPP

As discussed at the start of this chapter, mental imagery is a feature of human cognition. Just as traditional forms of CBT work by targeting clients' verbal thoughts, so too can treatment gain traction by targeting people's mental imagery. One key feature of mental imagery is that it has a powerful impact on emotion—something of particular relevance to BD. Moreover, a focus on mental imagery opens up the possibility that we can try out a range of new intervention techniques, such as rescripting imagery or creating adaptive positive imagery.

BD is a recurrent, severe, complex mental disorder, as discussed in Chapter 1, and it is generally treated with medication. But as also mentioned in that chapter, not all clients respond to current drug therapies; 50–60% of people with BD relapse within 1 year of recovery from an episode (Kessing et al., 2004). In addition, individuals with BD tend to experience residual anxiety and depressive symptoms throughout their lives, even between episodes of depression, mania, or hypomania (Judd et al., 2002). In view of that track record, and of the damaging effects the disorder has on clients and those close to them, new types of interventions tailored to the needs (and strengths) of this group are long overdue.

One potential development might be to examine the (at times) problematic mental imagery that we know exists in BD and to use imagery-focused CBT techniques to help stabilize mood (see the BAP guidelines; Goodwin et al., 2016). Again, we know that mood instability (moving between positive and negative mood) persists in BD, even when an individual is not experiencing full-blown mania or depression. Mental imagery can act as an "emotional amplifier" of mood states—anxiety, depression, and mania (Holmes, Geddes, et al., 2008)—and thus can exacerbate mood swings. People with BD can have vivid, distressing emotional imagery (e.g., of committing suicide; Hales et al., 2011) or imagery associated with manic mood states (e.g., of winning awards/buying expensive cars; Ivins et al., 2014). Furthermore, in Chapter 1, we have discussed the finding that people who score high on measures of bipolar character traits are more susceptible to developing negative intrusive imagery after a stressor (Malik et al., 2014). Therefore, finding ways to help clients reduce/ignore problematic imagery and/or to enhance adaptive imagery should contribute to improving mood stability in BD. Moreover, the potential benefits of working with imagery should also be relevant across any psychological difficulties (such as those discussed in Chapter 1) in which mental imagery affects emotion, not just BD.

With these ideas driving our efforts, we developed MAPP as a clinical psychology service for BD, within the psychiatrist-led Mood Disorders Clinic in Oxford, United Kingdom (Hales et al., 2018). The development of the approach has been an interdisciplinary endeavor, including input from clinical psychology, psychiatry, experimental psychology, neuroscience, and math. Psychological treatment innovation informed by mental health science is a team effort.

In MAPP, we provide extended psychological assessments and individual structured psychological treatments (described in detail in Part III) for clients with BD, based upon prinicples of CBT and professional standards of care. The treatment spans 10 sessions. After assessment, a clinician and client agree on a treatment target (e.g., social anxiety, trauma) that has an impact on the client's mood stability. In essence, the approach:

1. Targets problematic imagery associated with BD in general, and bipolar anxiety in particular (if present).
2. Uses imagery-based CBT techniques, such as those used for anxiety disorders (e.g., social anxiety disorder/social phobia).

The anxiety associated with BD is emphasized in part because of the high levels of comorbidity (up to 90%; Freeman et al., 2002; Merikangas et al., 2007). Moreover, as mentioned in Chapter 1, we know that the presence of anxiety in BD is a major contributor to poor functioning and a worse prognosis (Otto et al., 2006; Kroon et al., 2013), as well as to an increased suicide risk (Simon et al., 2007). However, as also discussed in Chapter 1, the medications traditionally used to manage anxiety can lead to a "manic switch" in people with BD (Baldessarini et al., 2013; Pacchiarotti et al., 2013). Therefore, addressing anxiety symptoms in psychological treatment may be critical to attaining full recovery in BD.

TESTING MAPP

Treatment innovation for BD has been hampered by a lack of techniques to target a hall-mark symptom: ongoing mood instability. Because of this, in developing MAPP we routinely monitored clients' mood symptoms via a daily and weekly self-report mood system. In this system (the True Colours system; for further information, see *https://oxfordhealth. truecolours.nhs.uk/www/en* and Miklowitz et al., 2012), clients sent in their mood ratings via short message service (i.e., text messaging) or email. Our key clinical outcome in testing MAPP was improvement in mood stability—namely, the symptom profile of mood scores before and after the psychological intervention. For example, repeated daily mood measurement (e.g., of depression) over a short time frame (1 month) provided data from which we created individual bipolar mood instability profiles/graphs. (In fact, using these profiles, clients can see and review their own progress over the course of treatment.) We also measured client satisfaction.

We tested the MAPP approach in a case series of 14 clients with BD (Holmes, Bonsall, et al., 2016). The results showed that weekly mood monitoring and treatment target data improved for the whole sample combined. In addition, mathematical time series analyses of the daily mood data, kept for 28 days pre- and posttreatment, demonstrated improvements in mood stability for 11 of the 14 clients (Holmes, Bonsall, et al., 2016). In addition, MAPP clients were highly satisfied with the intervention.

These findings offered preliminary support for this new imagery-focused treatment approach. Importantly, we found that daily measurement offers a description of individual mood instability in a clinically meaningful way, with clients finding it useful and encouraging to see graphs charting the progress they are making. Further research is warranted, and we hope that this book facilitates that endeavour.

CONCLUDING COMMENTS

BD can be a chronic and disabling mental illness, and we urgently need innovation in treatment approaches for it (whether these are pharmacological or psychological). MAPP shows promise as a treatment technique for improving mood stability in BD in a small number of sessions. The rest of this book details the general frame for implementing MAPP, and the assessment and treatment methods used in MAPP, in a clinician-friendly manualized format. As we emphasize throughout, while the original focus of MAPP was on working with mental imagery in BD, the techniques will be of use to clinicians working with a variety of psychological difficulties characterized by vivid mental images.

For further reading on mental imagery, we recommend the following: Pearson, Naselaris, Holmes, and Kosslyn (2015), for good coverage of the scientific background to mental imagery; Hackmann et al. (2011), for detailed descriptions of how to design and implement behavioral experiments; Holmes, Blackwell, Burnett Heyes, Renner, and Raes (2016), for a review of the role of mental imagery in depression; and Holmes, Geddes, Colom, and Goodwin (2008), for a review of imagery as an emotional amplifier in BD.

PART II
Overarching Principles and Basic Techniques

CHAPTER 3

The MAPP Therapeutic Ethos

As discussed in Chapter 1, BD arises from the interplay of numerous biological, psychological, and social factors whose relevance and roles may vary at different stages of the illness. Clinicians agree that there is no one specific presentation of BD. Research suggests that most people with BD will spend more time in depressed mood states than in mania or hypomania, but the profile of mood fluctuation varies widely among individuals (see Figure 3.1 for a mood profile typical of BD). In addition, many people with BD experience significant anxiety and other comorbid disorders, such as substance misuse.

As also discussed in Chapter 1, the NICE (2014) guidance for BD and the more recent BAP treatment guidelines (Goodwin et al., 2016) both underscore the importance of tailoring an intervention to the individual needs of each client, based on an individualized assessment and psychological formulation.

We designed the MAPP intervention with the NICE and BAP guidelines in mind. Our aim in developing MAPP was to do the following:

• Treat one imagery-related target that is clinically distressing or destabilizing and exacerbates symptoms, rather than attempting to address every aspect of the disorder. In comparatively complex populations, such as individuals with histories of childhood abuse (Steil, Jung, & Stangier, 2011) or refugees with complex PTSD (Arntz et al., 2013), imagery interventions have been shown to have clinical benefits beyond reduction of the target problematic imagery symptoms.

• Understand that the type of intervention and support needed by clients with BD is likely to change across the different phases of the illness. Thus we aimed to construct a therapy model that combines different integrated "modules" and offers a set of strategies to be used flexibly according to the various phases. Indeed, this approach may be more useful than offering separate interventions conceived in isolation, delivered only once and often focused on "firefighting" acute relapses.

• Provide a program that can be delivered alongside psychiatric intervention, including medication, with due sensitivity to client preferences. While not all clients with BD are under psychiatric care, a significant proportion of them are. MAPP is an approach that

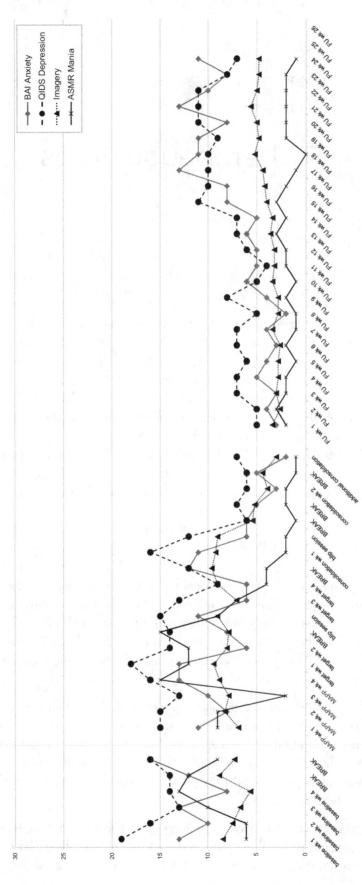

FIGURE 3.1. Example of a mood profile for a client with BD over the course of MAPP treatment. The crosses represent symptoms of mania, and the circles represent symptoms of depression. This person's symptoms of mania (measured by the Altman Self-Rating Mania Scale [ASRM]; Altman, Hedeker, Peterson, & Davis, 1997) started out at a subclinical level but varied a great deal during the early stages of treatment, becoming clinically significant at times. At the end of treatment, the manic symptoms varied much less, and they remained very low (subclinical) for 6 months. The client's symptoms of depression (measured by the Quick Inventory of Depressive Symptomatology [QIDS]; Rush et al., 2003) started out very high but were reduced to subclinical levels during the early stages of MAPP treatment. By the end of the follow-up (FU) period, they had begun to increase again (to just within the clinical range), though not to pretreatment levels of severity. BAI, Beck Anxiety Inventory.

24

works effectively in tandem with psychiatric and social care interventions. Liaison across disciplines to provide joined-up care is an integral part of the MAPP ethos (see also "Liaison with Other Mental Health Professionals," below.)

• Provide a service that acknowledges mood oscillations or "blips" as part of the long-term clinical picture of BD, and offers management of such "blips" within the context of the program.

• Provide an intervention that will improve overall mood stability, as well as reduce levels of anxiety and depression.

• Provide therapeutic input in a collaborative, transparent, and nonhierarchical way. Each therapist's thinking is shared with each client, and the client is encouraged to make his or her own decisions about therapy. In addition, in our MAPP case series, the MAPP manual was shared with each client from the outset.

• Provide therapeutic input in a curious way, modeling an experimental stance. It is hard to know which techniques will work well for each client. But even when things do not go well, as long as all ideas are introduced with an attitude of curiosity, the client and therapist will have learned something that will be of use as they move forward.

In the rest of the chapter, we give further information about some aspects of the MAPP therapeutic ethos: liaison with other mental health professionals; the use of cotherapists; and scaffolding the therapy to ensure that it stays on track.

LIAISON WITH OTHER MENTAL HEALTH PROFESSIONALS

Not all people living with BD come into contact with services; however, those who do are generally cared for within specialist mental health care services, including routine contact with a psychiatrist. In the United Kingdom, for example, the majority of people with BD currently receive psychiatric care alone, without access to psychological input. The MAPP approach is one that is complementary to medication and psychiatric input, and can be a useful adjunct to other, nonconcurrent psychological therapies.

Among the integral parts of the MAPP approach are regular liaison and collaboration with other mental health services involved in a client's care. These occur more often and to a greater extent than might be expected in routine clinical care. There are a number of reasons for this. First, as we have just said, MAPP is shaped by a collaborative, transparent, and nonhierarchical therapeutic approach. This approach also extends to relationships among professionals. Second, this approach means that mood oscillations or emerging risk issues can be managed quickly and safely, with the minimum disruption to the client. Third, information about effective strategies developed in the MAPP sessions are communicated to all members of a client's care team, so that this information can be revisited at a later date if the client has a relapse.

In our development and use of MAPP, we have engaged in close liaison with other mental health services at a number of time points during the program, Some of these contacts have been planned, and others have occurred in response to client need, as detailed below.

• At the point of referral, we have found it useful to have a discussion with the referrer. This has enabled us both to understand the nature of the referral and to underline that the MAPP approach does *not* represent an all-encompassing "cure" for BD, but rather tackles one distressing or destabilizing imagery-based target. We have also found it helpful to share information on how to describe and assess for clinically relevant imagery with our psychiatric colleagues—for example, by providing information sheets. (See Appendix 1 for the information sheet given to other professionals.)

• At the end of the assessment ("mapping") phase, a report is sent to the referrer, which outlines useful background information (such as a list of early warning signs indicated by the client, a timeline of mood episodes and relevant life events, and positive coping strategies). It also includes an assessment of imagery symptoms having an impact on mood. This report is written collaboratively with the client. It sets a clear focus for treatment and also provides an opportunity to communicate other information—such as difficulties with medication side effects—with the wider health care team.

• At the end of treatment, a further report is sent to the referrer. A key aspect of this report is to communicate the newly learned strategies and have these easily accessible for mental health workers involved in the client's care in the future. Our philosophy is that if the imagery-based strategies are made available to all care team members, the client can be encouraged to keep practicing the strategies in the future or to revisit them if they have been forgotten. To facilitate this, the imagery strategies are briefly described on the first page of the end-of-treatment report, alongside their impact on mood or anxiety, in order to be of practical use to all clinicians.

• In addition to the types of planned liaisons described above, communication takes place in response to a need to manage mood or risk issues. A distinct advantage of the MAPP approach is that therapists have access to mood-monitoring data from the beginning of MAPP. Therapists can thus detect mood deterioration through this data (and through direct contact in sessions) quickly and initiate appropriate action (medication reviews or increased support). This type of liaison can play an important role in preventing major bipolar episodes or relapses by signaling mood deterioration at early stages, when a combination of cognitive and behavioral strategies, medication adjustment, or other support may be enough to prevent mood from dramatically swinging up or down. Not only is this type of liaison and collaboration important to solve problematic short crises during therapy, but it also models a behavior that clients can then learn and acquire themselves to use independently in the future.

Case Example: Gillian

Gillian was a 30-year-old woman with a diagnosis of BD Type I who was pleased to have become pregnant with her first child. She had taken lithium for many years, and this had allowed her to reduce relapses and in particular prevent major manic episodes over the last 5 years. Nevertheless, she was concerned that her worries about possible risk for the fetus might push her toward suddenly stopping all medication. She had looked up lithium's safety profile on the internet, but remained unsure about it. She would have preferred to stop taking the drug but was worried about relapsing; however, she had not shared her concerns with her psychiatrist for fear that she might be put on something more sedative than lithium, as she had been in the past. These thoughts were fueling a mental state characterized by minor rapid swings between anxiety and elation about the pregnancy, with accompanying restlessness and mild hyperactivity. Happily, Gillian was able to share her preoccupations with her MAPP therapist.

The following steps were then put in place:

1. Gillian and the MAPP therapist discussed how to communicate Gillian's concerns to her psychiatrist, including dedicating part of the next therapy session to a brief joint meeting
2. The therapist and Gillian had a "blip" management session (see Chapter 4) in which they focused on trying to articulate and understand her specific anxieties about medication, and her fear of relapse and pregnancy. These worries were summarized in a brief letter to the mental health team, drafted together by Gillian and her therapist. Gillian also kept the letter at hand for her to use with any other clinician and significant others (such as her mother) who supported her during the pregnancy
3. Following the joint meeting, Gillian's psychiatrist agreed to reduce the dose of lithium for the first trimester, while Gillian would engage in a plan of cognitive and behavioral strategies that reinforced her capacity to recognize and control minimal signs of mood deterioration, including her sense of when to contact the psychiatrist to reintroduce medication.

COTHERAPISTS: "THE MORE, THE MERRIER"?

In developing the MAPP intervention, we typically had two therapists present in every session (sometimes with one therapist joining remotely via video conferencing). What struck us were some of the benefits that emerged—most notably how it increased the speed of training and supervising new colleagues in how to implement the therapeutic procedure, and how much our clients liked it.

In this section, we describe how multitherapist treatment worked in practice. However, while we greatly enjoyed the cotherapy model and can see some of its benefits, we think that it is unlikely to be an essential part of the intervention. This is a key point to make at the outset. Although using two therapists in MAPP sessions has some advantages, the quality of the treatment clients receive is likely to be no higher than that of treatment they would receive from a single therapist. In short, personnel constraints should not prohibit offering MAPP treatment.

Benefits of Having More Than One Therapist

In the development of MAPP, the two therapists present in any one session varied over time; the only rule was that each time, there must be one therapist present who had met with the client before. While this model represents a move away from the traditional client–therapist dyad, using this way of working has a number of advantages. In our experience, the cotherapist model can do the following:

1. Foster a collaborative, curious approach between therapists and client, partly by dint of flattening the hierarchy between the "professionals" and clients. This results in a stance of "We're all in this together . . . three heads, all trying to work out what will help."
2. Help all parties to keep each session on track and adhere to the agreed-upon agenda, particularly if clients are highly anxious or hypomanic.
3. Enable therapists to take a more reflective stance than is often possible in a dyadic client–therapist relationship. The therapists can explicitly provide feedback and reflections to each other in the session, which also models problem solving to the client.
4. Help to introduce different perspectives, interaction styles, and explanations to the client via the differences between the two therapists.
5. Be experienced by clients as *less* intense than a dyadic client–therapist relationship, which may be important, given that people with BD commonly describe interpersonal difficulties.
6. Increase the likelihood that the benefits of therapy will last and be generalized to other settings after it ends, by promoting multiple contexts and conversational partners.

Critical Points in the Cotherapy Model

There are several critical points to bear in mind for the model of "the more, the merrier" to work well:

1. Therapists must ensure that they model the nonhierarchical, collaborative approach in their stance toward *each other*, as well as toward the client.
2. In practice, the therapist dyad may often be made up of a more senior and more junior practitioner, or of practitioners from different professional backgrounds (e.g., a clinical psychologist and a psychiatrist). However, every attempt should be made to flatten any power differential between the two therapists in sessions.
3. The therapeutic ethos is of three *equal* individuals (two therapists and one client) being thoughtful and curious *together*, to map out the client's *present difficulties* and to find *creative solutions*.

What Does Cotherapy Look Like in MAPP?

For most clinicians, working with clients on a one-on-one basis is the norm, so the cotherapy model may take some getting used to. As we have stated, the model is explicitly nonhierarchical. Therapists are there to support each other and to form an equilateral triangle with the client: three equal partners collaborating in the tasks of therapy. One therapist may lead the session (e.g., by setting an agenda and taking a lead in addressing items on it), while the other has the role of "scaffolding" the session, ensuring that the session remains on track, and reflecting back and summarizing important information.

How Do Therapists and Clients Feel about the Cotherapy Model?

MAPP clinicians often report that "the more, the merrier" is a particularly useful model. Here are some points they raise:

1. If one of the therapists has not been present in every session, this can be used to the advantage of the therapy. This cotherapist might open a session as follows: "For my benefit, as I was not in the last session, could you summarize for me what you've been working on?" Responding to this question not only updates the clinician who was not present, but also gives the client an opportunity to summarize the work he or she has done, and to begin to consolidate learning and be the person leading and taking responsibility for the work. (During the MAPP case series, we often swapped in different cotherapists. Although we did this primarily for logistical reasons, we found that introducing a "new pair of eyes" was refreshing for all and was received positively.)

2. If the lead therapist is getting stuck in the therapy session, he or she can use the other therapist to help reflect on what's happening. The lead therapist can explicitly say, for example: "I notice that it seems we are finding it harder to stick to our agenda this week than we have done before, and I'm wondering if you have any ideas about what's happening and what we should do." The other therapist can then introduce new perspectives and model a curious stance to overcoming the barrier.

3. It can also be helpful for cotherapists to be frank with the client about being unsure of what to do next in a session, and to work together as a team to decide how to proceed—for example, by consulting the therapy manual. This openness models a curious, nonhierarchical, and collaborative approach and encourages a problem-solving stance.

What is it like for a client to be sitting in a room with not one, but two therapists? Generally, we have found that clients rate their experiences as overwhelmingly positive. Here are some representative comments clients made about the model when we conducted our audit of the pilot clinical service:

"Having cotherapists is an inspirational idea."

"The conversation always seemed to kind of flow really easily. . . . [There's] something about flow, rather than about a binary, one-to-one relationship."

"[I felt] as if I was part of an ongoing inquiry of theirs which mattered to them, as if I was contributing something, as if every exchange meant something to all of us because it was a genuine conversation."

"Whereas in the counseling scenario you sometimes feel quite pressurized and there is no one else there to see, there is something about having someone else there to see what is happening that is actually quite helpful."

Explaining "the More, the Merrier" to Clients

Despite the positive feedback noted above, prior to beginning therapy clients are often curious or a little anxious about having two therapists in the room. It can therefore be helpful to brief them. One of the therapists may want to use an explanation along the lines of this example:

> "There are a few things about MAPP that may differ from psychology or psychiatry appointments you've had before. First, you will have noticed that there are two therapists here. This is because, in our experience, we find that it's really helpful to be able to put three heads together rather than just two, to think about things in different ways and from different viewpoints. Our clients have said that although they might find this a little unusual at first, it is something that they tend to get used to quickly and really value."

SCAFFOLDING THERAPY

Studies demonstrate that people with BD may display a range of cognitive difficulties, such as concentration or remembering things (Malhi et al., 2007). Traditionally, these impairments have been viewed as being associated with depressed or (hypo)manic moods. However, in the past decade, neuropsychological research has shown that there is persistent cognitive impairment in BD even in periods of euthymia (Martínez-Arán et al., 2004). Areas that are particularly affected include attention, memory, and executive functions. Another area in which functioning may also be impaired is the perception of time (Mahlberg, Kienast, Bschor, & Adli, 2008).

In the therapy room, cognitive deficits may be manifested as trouble in:

- Focusing.
- Sustaining attention.
- Remembering learning from previous sessions.
- Remembering any homework.
- Putting learning into practice outside of sessions.
- Organizing thoughts (e.g., having a list of topics that the client wants to discuss, or prioritizing what to talk about).
- Remembering when the next appointment is.
- Staying on one topic for very long.

Scaffolding Techniques

In MAPP, we use the term "scaffolding" to describe techniques used to compensate for cognitive impairments. By using scaffolding techniques, we aim to support clients to engage in the MAPP interventions as fully as possible. In practice, this means that in MAPP the therapists are much more proactive than in "standard" CBT in ensuring that the clients attend sessions and are able to benefit from the therapy.

The following scaffolding techniques are integral parts of the MAPP approach, running through all mapping, treatment, follow-up, and "blip" management sessions:

- A text message appointment reminder is sent the day before any arranged MAPP appointment.
- A letter of confirmation is provided of any future appointment slots agreed upon in person.
- At the start of every session, a written agenda is agreed upon between therapists and client, and placed in a visible position for the duration of the session. (See Appendix 2 for agendas for all 10 sessions of the MAPP protocol.)
- An agreement is reached between therapists and client that when the session wanders off target, one of the therapists will intervene to bring the focus back to the agreed-upon agenda.
- Visual memory aids are used to help consolidate key pieces of learning (e.g., writing strategies on picture postcards, using visual metaphors as reminders; see the case of Jenny below for further details).
- When the therapists and client are deciding on homework tasks, attention is paid to how the client can remember to do them—for example, by setting alarms or reminders on a mobile phone, putting reminder notes in prominent places in the client's home, or asking a significant other to help remind him or her.
- "Blueprints" of learning at the end of the therapy take the form of videos rather than traditional written records. In CBT, blueprints are summaries of what the client has learned over therapy, and they normally involve a plan for what to do if similar difficulties arise in the future. Our hope is that when clients make these blueprints in video format, they will be more likely to remember what they have learned and to view the blueprints in the future. (There is no need for expensive recording/viewing equipment; mobile phone recordings, photographs, or drawings will serve the same purpose as videos.) The making of blueprints is covered in detail in Chapter 12.

Rationale for Scaffolding

Some clients initially resist the whole idea of scaffolding techniques, because they may feel that these are infantilizing or disempowering. With a solid alliance, a therapist can work through this hesitation. It helps to provide such a client with a clear rationale. Here is one possible way of presenting such a rationale:

"People with bipolar disorder sometimes find it difficult to remember appointments, or have problems with staying focused on one topic, or perhaps have trouble being organized. Does that sound familiar to you at all? One of the things we do in the MAPP approach is to try to do specific things both in and out of the sessions to provide some 'scaffolding.' We find that this helps our clients to attend sessions, to focus on the most important topics in sessions, and to remember the learning from these sessions better.

"Some of the things we will do are to text you a reminder of your appointment the day before each session; make sure at the beginning of each session that we have a shared agenda of the most important things to cover; and help you to work out strategies so that you can remember what we've discussed outside of sessions—for example, by taking home postcards with key points written on them. Does that sound like it would be useful?"

Case Examples

Example 1: Jenny

Jenny had a diagnosis of BD Type II and generalized anxiety disorder. She reported that when she noticed any small change in mood, she would interpret this as a sign that she was going to have a serious mood episode, and that this interpretation would result in high anxiety. In response to this anxiety, she would withdraw from others and on occasion drink excessively, which had the effect of intensifying any mood symptoms.

In the MAPP intervention, one of the things we did was to encourage Jenny to devise a visual metaphor to remind herself that she could "ride out" small changes in mood without getting caught up in an anxiety cycle. Jenny created an image of a boat going up and down on the sea—rising and falling with the waves, but not getting swept away by them. She was encouraged to bring this image to mind when she found herself feeling anxious about mood changes. To scaffold this strategy further—that is, to help herself to remember it and put it into practice—Jenny drew a postcard of the sea, wrote some prompts on the back of it, and stuck it on her fridge door at home where she could see it often.

Example 2: Sira

Sira had a diagnosis of BD Type I and social anxiety disorder/social phobia. The main focus of the MAPP intervention with her was to rescript an intrusive image of herself doing badly in a social situation. She reported that the "antidote" (rescripted) image of herself doing well in a social situation was very useful for her to practice, particularly before she attended social events. However, she struggled to remember to practice this antidote image outside of sessions. Following a discussion in one session, Sira decided that she would set an alert on her phone each morning to prompt her to bring to mind the antidote image on a daily basis. Once this strategy was devised, Sira practiced using the antidote image regularly, which resulted in a corresponding decrease in social anxiety.

Hints and Tips for Using the Cotherapy Model to Scaffold Sessions

Some clients find it very difficult to stay focused on one topic, particularly if they are very anxious or experiencing (hypo)manic symptoms. In situations such as these, it can be helpful to explicitly and openly assign roles for the two therapists. One therapist leads the session and provides the intervention; the second therapist keeps track of the agenda and the session time. Specifically, the second therapist's role is to (1) notice when the session starts to move away from the agreed-upon target and point out to the others that this has happened; (2) keep emphasizing the importance of coming back to the agreed-upon target; and (3) keep track of time so that each agenda item can be sufficiently covered during the session.

CLIENT REFLECTIONS ON THE MAPP THERAPEUTIC ETHOS

The following are direct quotes from MAPP clients who were asked for feedback at the end of treatment, and are used with their permission. They reflect the attitude or ethos that runs through MAPP, for both the client and the therapist—of being collaborative, curious, and experimental when working with mental imagery.

"No one is perfect, and nothing works all the time. There are no hard-and-fast rules. But experiment. The more you try, the more chance of finding something that will work for you. Don't be afraid to explore and take control. The journey is about you. Yes, the unknown is scary, but you'll never know if you don't try."

"Be honest with [the therapists]—pretending something has worked won't get you anywhere. When they ask you to try doing things, do them, and take them seriously. Not everything you try will work, and that is just fine. My MAPP journey was neither a short nor an easy process, but it worked for me. We started with developing specific strategies focused on specific issues I was having trouble with, and it grew from there. We tried to identify where the problem was and how we might tackle it, and as we tried things, we learned more about the problem, and so were more able to create strategies that worked."

"Let yourself be surprised. The most unusual, unexpected, and surprising elements of the sessions will be the most insightful. Take home with you the impressions and thoughts that the sessions and discussions will bring to the surface. They will bear fruits in good time, mostly in the days following. Take the suggested techniques seriously, even if they appeared strange or bizarre at first, and take your time to give them a fair chance to work. But be discerning; not everything will suit you, and it's right you should find what best works for you. [Also,] don't expect this to be immediate; much trial and error is required. Don't let temporary disappointment put you off the overall process."

CONCLUDING COMMENTS

In this chapter, we have first outlined the key features of the therapeutic ethos of the MAPP intervention. Then we have given more details about some particular aspects of the approach: the liaison with other mental health professionals, the use of cotherapists, and the scaffolding of the therapy structure. In the next chapter, we go on to discuss how to monitor and cope with fluctuations in mood and how to encourage clients to be kind to themselves.

CHAPTER 4

Mood Monitoring, "Blip" Management, and Being Kind to Oneself

In this chapter, we outline three basic techniques or principles that run through all of the work we do with MAPP clients: mood monitoring, "blip" management, and being kind to oneself.

MOOD MONITORING

"Mood monitoring" refers to the regular (daily or weekly) recording of mood by clients, using either idiosyncratic or standardized measures. Mood monitoring is integral to the MAPP process. A key requirement of entering the MAPP case series was that clients had to be willing to complete weekly self-report measures of depression (the Quick Inventory of Depressive Symptomatology or QIDS; Rush et al., 2003), mania (the Altman Self-Rating Mania Scale or ASRM; Altman, Hedeker, Peterson, & Davis, 1997), and anxiety (the Beck Anxiety Inventory or BAI; Beck, Brown, Epstein, & Steer, 1988). These measures were completed either online or in paper-and-pencil format.

Mood monitoring is a key part of most psychoeducational interventions for BD (see Colom & Vieta, 2006, for a list). There is evidence that mood monitoring alone may result in improvement in depression scores for clients with a diagnosis of BD Type II (Bopp et al., 2010), even in the absence of any further therapeutic intervention. A key benefit of mood monitoring is that it can quickly alert a client and therapist to any significant changes in mood (or "blips"), so strategies can be implemented to manage mood before a potential mood episode becomes entrenched.

When clients rate their moods regularly, their therapists can use this information to create graphs of mood that can be reviewed with the clients in their sessions. In Oxford, United Kingdom, Professor John Geddes and colleagues at the University of Oxford have developed a system called True Colours (*https://oxfordhealth.truecolours.nhs.uk/www/en*), mentioned in Chapter 2. True Colours allows a client to fill in mood questionnaires online and view the scores in an individualized chart.

There are lots of online apps now that clients can use to monitor their moods, but it is also fine to use paper-based questionnaires. These can be completed by clients in or before sessions, and the resulting data can be plotted directly on a paper-based graph, which the clients and therapists can then review collaboratively. Again, mood monitoring alone can have a beneficial effect on mood stability, but when mood-monitoring data is reviewed with clients in sessions, it can have a number of additional therapeutic functions, as outlined below.

Overview of the Technique

The precise details of mood monitoring will vary according to which systems are available locally, as discussed earlier. However, during the MAPP trial, we used hard copies of individual clients' mood-monitoring data (in the form of graphs of their scores on weekly measures) for a variety of purposes:

- Alerting clients and therapists to any recent changes in mood that might signal the beginning of an episode of (hypo)mania or depression.
- Helping clients to identify triggers for mood changes.
- Noticing patterns in mood fluctuation (e.g., at particular times of year).
- Combating biased memory recall of emotional states (see the case example of Campbell, below).
- Monitoring the impact of any intervention strategy.
- Reviewing progress over the course of the MAPP sessions.

Please note that although we would consider it good practice to have a brief look at the mood-monitoring graphs in every MAPP session, it is not necessary to review the data *in significant detail* with clients in every single session, unless this is felt to be important in terms of the session agenda or issues arising through discussion.

Rationale for Mood Monitoring

The rationale for mood monitoring can be explained to clients in the following way:

"Studies suggest that just monitoring mood alone can have a beneficial effect on stabilizing mood. When you take a moment each week to monitor and record your mood, it can help you to notice 'blips' (points when your mood starts to change) more quickly, so you can do something about it before the mood sets in and becomes entrenched. When you monitor your mood over a period of time, it can also make you aware of any patterns in mood fluctuations—for example, around stressful events at work or college. This can then encourage you to plan strategies to help you manage stressors on the horizon that may have an impact on your mood. In addition, in our sessions, we can review your graphs together to monitor your progress and make sure that the things we are working on together are having a stabilizing effect on your mood. Does that make sense? Do you have any questions about that?"

Case Example: Campbell

Campbell had a diagnosis of BD Type I, social anxiety disorder/social phobia, and panic disorder. During his MAPP assessment, he experienced a significant increase in symptoms of depression, triggered coincidentally by difficulties in a close relationship. During the third MAPP session, he reported: "For the past few years, I've pretty much always been depressed, and I know that I just won't be able to get out of it; there's nothing I can do." This belief was associated with high levels of hopelessness and suicidal ideation.

The MAPP therapists introduced the concept of "state-dependent memory" to Campbell. That is, when we are in a particular mood state, we are much more likely to remember other times when we have been in that same mood state. This can have the effect, for example, of making us believe we have always felt low, when in reality this has not been the case. Campbell understood this concept. The MAPP therapists and Campbell then looked together at his graph of mood symptoms. He was able to notice that although there had been times in the past 3 months when he had experienced episodes of depression, he had also had periods of comparatively stable, euthymic mood. From looking at the graph, he also noticed that the episodes of depression he had experienced *had* resolved; that is, "I was able to come out of them."

Looking at Campbell's mood-monitoring chart in session with him helped him to develop a new perspective on his current experience of depression: "When I feel depressed, it seems like I have always felt this way and the depression will just continue going on forever, but actually that is not true. Looking at the graph reminds me that although I may have times when I feel depressed, they do not last forever, and I just need to hang on to that fact and ride them out, rather than giving up hope."

Hints and Tips for Increasing Motivation for/ Adherence to Mood Monitoring

Most MAPP therapists clearly set out the rationale for mood monitoring, so clients will be aware of the potential benefits of doing it regularly from the outset of their sessions. Nonetheless, there may be times when clients do not feel fully engaged with the mood-monitoring process. Below is a list of common difficulties that clients may experience with mood monitoring, along with suggested strategies for therapists to help improve the clients' motivation and adherence to the process.

• *A client reports that he or she intends to complete the measures, but forgets to fill them in.* Therapists can use "scaffolding" techniques to help the client remember to complete the measures—for example, by making a plan to put up reminders in prominent places, or agreeing on a particular time of each day to complete measures so as to get into a habit. Therapists may also wish to set up other external reminders. For example, in our case series we sent text messages to clients on an agreed-upon day and time each week, prompting them to complete measures. It may also be possible to negotiate with clients to have them arrive 10 minutes before their sessions begin and complete measures then.

- *A client feels that the measures "don't capture what I'm really going through."* Most therapists agree that mood measures can sometimes be "blunt instruments" and do not capture every aspect of individual experience. The client should nevertheless be encouraged to continue completing the mood measures, as they build up a picture of long-term variations in mood stability and can be very valuable for the client. However, it is also helpful to have an open discussion about whether additional standardized or idiosyncratic measures could be used to capture experiences that are particularly relevant to clients. Such a measure could simply be a single item. For example, in the True Colours system (Miklowitz et al., 2012), clients are able to rate a particular behavioral measure that they feel is related to mood, such as number of cigarettes smoked or number of hours spent in the company of others each day.

- *A client reports that "focusing on my mood makes me feel worse."* The therapists can explore with the client whether this is actually the case (as it sometimes is), or whether the client is avoiding mood monitoring because of a belief that it may make him or her feel worse. The therapists can reassure the client that although it can be scary to think about how he or she is feeling, the long-term benefits of doing so can be great. The client can be encouraged not to spend too much time thinking about the answers on the measures, but rather to fill them in quickly. It might be helpful for the client to plan to complete the measures directly before a pleasant or absorbing activity (to avoid rumination), or outside of activities or responsibilities that may increase anxiety (e.g., work).

"BLIP" MANAGEMENT

The key feature of BD is chronic mood instability; therefore, management of problematic mood "blips" is a key skill that is modeled and taught over the course of the MAPP intervention. "Blips" is a term often used by clients themselves to describe minor but significant shifts in mood (in any direction); they may be warning signs of further mood instability, or may simply be temporary states that will right themselves if managed appropriately. (We knew it would be important to focus on managing these shifts within our treatment module, and so we adopted the term "blips" because clients were comfortable with it.)

Overview of the Technique

The aims of a "blip" management session are (1) to help the client identify immediate strategies to implement to help stabilize mood, and (2) to increase the client's perceived sense of control over the mood symptoms. "Blip" management emphasizes practical strategies and self-care to help the client get back on track. As much as possible, clients should be encouraged to use strategies they know have helped them in the past (e.g., talking to a friend or parent, limiting alcohol, promoting good sleep, using imagery techniques learned in therapy), rather than developing a completely new repertoire of strategies, as the former are likely to be easier to implement. In essence, we try to encourage a client not to see a "blip" as catastrophic; we emphasize that experiencing a shift in mood like this does not have to mean that the client is going to fall into a full-blown manic or depressive state. We encourage the client not to panic or to become disheartened, but to make a plan to cope and to get back to how they were before. A typical "blip" management intervention will include the following ingredients (for more details about these, see "Description of Steps," below):

1. Liaison with psychiatry/general practitioner.
2. Framing of mood symptoms as a "blip."
3. (Re)instatement of behavioral routines that promote mood stability.
4. Identification of strategies that have been effective in managing previous mood episodes.
5. Education regarding the importance of a self-compassionate stance.
6. Development of a written action plan for "blip" management.
7. Additional support to implement the plan via telephone/face-to-face check-ins with therapist(s).

Rationale for "Blip" Management

The rationale for focusing on "blip" management can be explained to clients by saying something like this:

> "From what you're saying, it seems that you're having a bit of a 'blip' in your mood at the moment. That's OK; these are things we will all experience from time to time. The good thing is that this 'blip' has happened during the course of our MAPP sessions, so we have a great opportunity to work together now to practice how you can put in place strategies to get you back on track, which you can then use again for any future 'blips.' How does that sound to you?"

Description of Steps

Liaison with Psychiatry/General Practitioner

- Communication and joint work with our psychiatric/mental health team/general practitioner/other significant colleagues are considered integral parts of the MAPP approach.
- Depending on the severity of a client's mood "blip," different levels of liaison may be deemed necessary.
- As MAPP therapists, we make it explicit to clients from the outset that we work jointly with our psychiatric colleagues, and that we exchange information and communicate with them to ensure high standards of client care.

Framing of Mood Symptoms as a "Blip"

- Clients will tend to be alert to small changes in mood and can misinterpret these as signs of a full-blown mood episode rather than simply a "blip." The clients may then, for example, become hopeless and feel helpless to manage their mood, giving up any helpful routines and thereby worsening their mood. Thus a "blip" that could have been "ridden out" can become a full-blown mood episode.

- Because of this, MAPP therapists educate their clients that a "blip" is often just that and will resolve with some attention and implementation of mood management strategies.

- Clients have frequently found it useful to create a visual metaphor of being able to "ride out" the ups and downs of their moods—for example, imagining a boat or buoy on the ocean, calmly rising and falling with the waves and remaining safe and intact.

(Re)instatement of Behavioral Routines That Promote Mood Stability

- The therapists assess whether regular behavioral routines (sleep–wake cycles, regular mealtimes, regular exercise, etc.) are being adhered to. Typically, these behavioral routines become disrupted during a "blip."

- Clients should be encouraged to plan regular behavioral routines and stick to these (e.g., to go to bed each night and to get up each morning at the same time, even if this is hard to do; to eat something regularly, three times a day, even if their appetite is poor).

Identification of Strategies That Have Been Effective in Managing Previous Mood Episodes

- Discussion of previous "blips" and how these were resolved can help clients to identify strategies that they have found useful in the past for mood management. It can be helpful to look at a client's individual mood-monitoring graphs with him or her, to help foster these reflections.

- During the MAPP assessment sessions, a client should have identified a list of "positive coping strategies" for mood management, which will be detailed in the report. It is useful to refer back to this report with the client and discuss whether he or she is currently using any of these coping strategies. It is common for clients to notice that over time, these strategies have slipped from their regular routines.

Education Regarding the Importance of a Self-Compassionate Stance

- The importance of self-compassion and self-care during times of difficulty should be particularly emphasized in "blip" management sessions. Therapists will generally frame self-compassion as "being kind to oneself." (See also the section on "Being Kind to Oneself," below, and the discussion in Chapter 5 of how to use chair work from schema therapy to promote self-compassion.)

- Previous MAPP clients have commented that although they are happy looking after other people, they are less good at giving the same care and attention to themselves. The following metaphor has been helpful in emphasizing the need to prioritize oneself first before attending to others' needs:

  > "During the safety announcements on airplanes, there is a part where they talk about what to do if there is a drop in the air pressure in the cabin. The stewards will say that oxygen masks will drop from the ceiling, and that you should secure your own mask before helping others. Why do you think that is?"

Development of a Written Action Plan for "Blip" Management

- Once a plan for "blip" management has been developed with the client, this should be written down for the client to take away and refer back to. The format can be tailored to the individual; for example, it could take the form of a postcard that can be carried around in a bag or stuck to a wall.

- MAPP therapists always make a record of the "blip" management plan and then send this out to clients in the form of a letter (or an email) in case the clients lose their copy. Significant others (e.g., family, friends, or even the care team) may be able to help reinforce a "blip" management plan—although this will need to be agreed upon in advance.

Additional Support to Implement the Plan Via Telephone/Face-to-Face
Check-Ins with Therapist(s)

- A limited number of additional face-to-face sessions or between-session phone calls can be agreed upon, to help support the client in implementing the "blip" management plan.

Case Example: Juan

Juan had a diagnosis of BD Type II and OCD. He had engaged with the MAPP intervention well and had shown improvements in mood stability and anxiety over the course of the treatment sessions. During the follow-up period, he encountered a particularly stressful situation when his best friends decided to divorce, and he felt as a result that he would lose one or the other of them as a friend. During the period of the divorce court case, Juan was repeatedly asked to help his friends with child care, as their son attended the same nursery school as Juan's daughter. Every time he had to drop his friend's son back at their house, Juan anticipated witnessing another argument between his friends, and his levels of anxiety and depression spiked sharply.

MAPP delivered four "blip" management sessions via telephone over the course of the court case. These consisted of appointments lasting approximately 30 minutes each with one of the MAPP therapists involved in Juan's treatment. Juan reported that he found it helpful for the therapist to help him identify what he needed to do to get back on track during the time when he "could not think clearly." In particular, he valued the therapist's structuring information and strategies for him, and summarizing this in a written plan, which was emailed to him directly following each phone call and then also sent out in the form of a letter.

Juan had a tendency to deny his own needs and focus on supporting others, and the therapist worked hard to emphasize the need for self-care as a key "blip" management strategy. In subsequent feedback, Juan stated that this self-care component had been important in getting back on track: "I've learned that if I sometimes can't help my friends and take time to look after myself, they will still be my friends, and the world is not going to end."

Following these "blip" management sessions, Juan's mood returned to a more stable pattern, and he managed well the stressors associated with witnessing his friends' breakup and supporting them, as well as remaining friends with both of them after the divorce.

Hints and Tips on Therapist Stance in "Blip" Management Sessions: Socratic or Directive?

CBT emphasizes collaboration, and therapists will generally tend to take a "Socratic" stance in sessions. A Socratic stance is one in which a therapist uses open questioning to help a client uncover information, investigate issues, and develop understanding. That is, the therapist is not telling the client what to do or providing direct guidance; rather, the therapist facilitates the client's own learning and self-discovery. However, previous MAPP clients have reported that it can be helpful for MAPP therapists to be quite directive during "blip" management sessions. Executive skills (including the ability to plan for the future) can be reduced during mood episodes, and so it may be hard for clients to generate a plan for themselves without a good deal of scaffolding and other support (see Chapter 3 for a discussion of scaffolding).

A rule of thumb is for MAPP therapists is to start by identifying "blip" management strategies Socratically with clients, thereby modeling a problem-solving approach. However, if it is difficult for clients to generate strategies, then a more directive approach is likely to be indicated. In our MAPP sessions during the case series, if the therapists judged that a client needed a more directive approach, they explained that to the client explicitly by saying something like this:

"I can see that it is quite hard for you to know what will help your mood at the moment. That's all right; when mood gets wobbly, it can be hard to think clearly. If it's OK, I'm going to be more directive than usual and suggest some strategies to use to help you get back on track. How does that sound?"

Client Reflection on Mood Monitoring and "Blip" Management

Below is an example of what a MAPP client might say when asked for feedback at the end of treatment, regarding the usefulness of learning to monitor and control moods.

"Since my therapy stopped and life went on, many things have changed. But MAPP taught me that [an important thing is] continuing to experiment with the techniques I discovered in therapy . . . and I have carried on with using them and (when needed) adapting them, so they continue to fit as things change over time. One of my favorite aspects of MAPP is this: It's like having an interesting conversation between you and the therapists, so actually you are the one actively developing the skills and strategies yourself too, and that means you continue doing it even after the therapy. It's a joint dialogue where you learn about what suddenly stops you in your tracks and how to change that and go on. I used to be paralyzed by the fear that too much could go wrong. Now I have strategies, and those fears have dissipated. I have become aware of what I can do in a given situation to stay well, and this has given me much better control over my mood. For me, it was definitely a worthwhile journey."

BEING KIND TO ONESELF

In general, teaching our clients ways of being kind to themselves is a great idea. But why do we think it is particularly important in working with people who have BD? The research literature tells us that some of the life experiences and personality characteristics that are often present in BD may contribute to the development of difficulties in taking care of and being compassionate toward oneself.

As we all know, BD is a recurrent, often chronic, and severe illness, which has the potential to impair several domains of everyday life. Yet it may also include episodes when clients act in a disinhibited manner, during hypomanic or manic phases. This may lead clients to feel ashamed about their behavior during these phases. In addition, we know that there is a high prevalence of past trauma in the histories of clients with BD (Simon et al., 2004, 2007), which can be associated with chronic feelings of shame and/or guilt. Furthermore, chronic conditions and a history of abuse or neglect have both been linked to low levels of self-compassion (Goldberg & Garno, 2005). Finally, evidence suggests that BD may be associated with traits such as perfectionism (Scott, Stanton, Garland, & Ferrier, 2000), unstable self-esteem (Knowles et al., 2007), and goal striving (Alloy et al., 2012), any of which can further reduce the ability to be kind to oneself.

In our experience, when clients have low levels of self-compassion, these tend to be manifested in one or more of the following ways:

- Imagery that contains themes centered on threat and/or self-criticism.
- An emotion regulation style that favors responding tvo negative situations by engaging in goal achievement activities (which are often excessively ambitious), rather than engaging in self-soothing activities. In addition, for people with BD, an excessive focus on goal achievement also potentially runs the risk of escalating (hypo)manic behaviors and symptoms.
- Overly negative or overly positive (rather than balanced) imagery related to self.
- Difficulties in engaging in therapeutic strategies that involve being kind to oneself.

These tendencies can then lessen the clients' ability or willingness to develop new strategies to help deal with anxiety, mood fluctuations, or other problematic symptoms. In particular, we have found that if clients adopt a self-critical stance, they are more likely to struggle to accept the inevitable obstacles and difficulties that arise when new skills and behaviors are being tested through therapy. In addition, once therapy is over, they are likely to find it harder to keep practicing and further developing what they have learned.

Thus a key facet of the MAPP treatment involves encouraging all clients to take on and foster attitudes and behaviors showing kindness toward, compassion for, and acceptance of themselves, across all stages of the therapy.

Overview of the Technique

Below, we describe several interventions that MAPP therapists have found helpful in enabling clients to develop a compassionate stance toward themselves during therapy.

Self-Compassionate and Balanced Positive Imagery

As part of either developing positive imagery or counteracting troublesome, intrusive negative imagery, clients can be encouraged to integrate elements of self-care and kindness into their images (see also Chapter 10). Examples of images our clients have used include having a warm bath, sitting down and having a cup of tea, someone else being caring or soothing toward them, and buying themselves a small treat (a plant, a cake). Clients are encouraged to try to use all of the senses when creating their images; olfactory (smell) and tactile images can be particularly powerful in adding to a sense of comfort or safety. When clients have long-held self-critical or self-punishing attitudes, *imagining* looking after themselves may act as an important precursor to actually being able to carry out a self-care action. For these clients, trying immediately to *behave* in a self-compassionate way may feel too overwhelming or risky.

The Perfect Nurturer

A useful technique based on compassion-focused therapy protocols is called "the perfect nurturer" (Lee, 2005). It involves helping a client to generate an image of a nurturing figure (someone or something, either real or imaginary) that the client can bring to mind and use in a variety of contexts. The client and therapist work together to develop a written description of the perfect nurturer. This might include how the nurturer looks, smells, sounds, and feels. The person/thing will also possess the qualities of acceptance, warmth, strength of mind, wisdom, genuineness, and hope. The nurturer is often a known or idealized person, but for some it can be an entity, an animal, or even a fictional place. After generating and refining a mental image of the perfect nurturer in sessions with the therapist, the client can then practice using the image when needed, to engender feelings of being soothed and nurtured (Lee & James, 2012).

Self-Soothing Activities

The therapist can explore with the client whether the client engages in any activities or behaviors that produce a sense of being calm, being taken care of, or "being OK." These might include talking to a friend, having a warm bath, or listening to music. These can come to light during the "positive coping strategies" part of the initial assessment sessions (see Chapter 6) or as part of later "blip" management sessions.

Chair Work to Overcome Self-Criticism

A technique called "chair work" (adapted from Gestalt and schema therapy) can be used to develop a kind and accepting stance toward oneself, particularly when clients struggle to recognize and acknowledge their own self-criticism (Arntz & Jacob, 2013). The therapist and client first identify the self-critical voice, and then can role-play adopting different attitudes and stances toward themselves. This technique can be particularly helpful when self-criticism tends to be triggered by the same types of situation or interactions with others. See Chapter 5 for more details on chair work.

Rationale for Being Kind to Oneself

The rationale for being kind to oneself can be explained to clients in the following way:

"When dealing with difficult situations, we all tend to adopt different styles of responding. These can generally be grouped into three categories.

"First, sometimes we focus on the negative aspects of the situation—on potential risks and negative outcomes—and decide to protect ourselves by avoiding a situation or by thinking about all of the things that we have done wrong (perhaps so that we can do better next time).

"Second, sometimes we respond by setting another goal, perhaps an even harder one, and engaging actively in achieving it—trying extremely hard to do our best, and perhaps putting ourselves under even more stress or pressure.

"Third, sometimes we recognize that we just need to give ourselves a break, be forgiving and understanding, and just take care of ourselves in order to feel better.

"Some people, especially if they have experienced many difficulties in their lives, find it hard to actually take some time out and take care of themselves. This is a shame, because addressing our difficulties by accepting the present, doing something soothing, and simply being self-compassionate can be so important in helping mood stay stable.

"Do you think this would apply to you? I have noticed that when things go wrong, you often respond by [description of the client's specific reaction]. How would you feel about exploring ways to take a kind stance toward yourself when things get hard?"

Case Examples

Example 1: Khaled

Khaled had a diagnosis of BD Type II. Even when his mood was relatively stable, he would continue to experience significant anxiety, often related to stressful situations in his job in a call center. Khaled experienced intrusive images of the inbox on his computer signaling how many phone calls were on hold for him to pick up; these images kept him from sleeping, which left him tired at work the following day. He also reported having intrusive images before meetings with his boss. In these, he would see his boss with a "giant mouth" talking and talking about how bad his performance was; it felt as if the mouth could devour him, and he could not even make sense of the words coming out of it. Recurrent themes embedded in his negative imagery were the sense of not being good enough for his position, and a belief that he constantly had to prove that he deserved it. He would berate himself for always struggling and (in his perception) failing in his work.

In contrast, Khaled had a loving relationship with his partner, David. During therapy, he engaged in an imagery rescripting exercise in which he first imagined the inbox full of incoming calls, and then turned his mind to imagining walking in the park, hand in hand with David. This resulted in his feeling much calmer and brought with it a sense of being loved and capable.

Following this exercise, Khaled acknowledged that always questioning whether he was doing well enough was not actually contributing to his doing better in his job, and in fact kept his anxiety levels high. Khaled was also encouraged to explore how he responded to David if David was worried about something at work or in his social life. He realized that often he would simply give him a hug or suggest a trip to a café or pub as a treat. He realized that trying to adopt this attitude to himself—to look after himself when stressed, rather than beat himself up and work even harder—might well be much more beneficial for him too.

Example 2: Mila

Mila had a diagnosis of BD Type I with onset in her early 20s, when she had just started dental school. Despite having had to take time off from her studies, she had managed to graduate and was now training to become an orthodontist. Mila also suffered from a mild form of arthritis, an inflammatory disease that needed regular medical checks and required her to do regular physical therapy exercises. She would often forget to attend her appointments and to do the exercises, relying on the fact that being a health care professional herself, she would recognize well enough if a "real" intervention was needed.

During the assessment phase, Mila realized that a worsening of the arthritis symptoms (she would feel stiff and have mild persistent pain at the end of the day) would often precede minor mood swings of both elation and depression. She was then encouraged by her therapist to discuss what she would prescribe to one of her relatives who suffered from similar problems. As a result, Mila introduced the following rule among her mood-monitoring and "blip" management strategies: that whenever her arthritis symptoms got even just slightly worse, she would take half a day off work, do her nails, and watch a DVD box set on her television. After adopting this strategy for a period of 2 months, Mila noticed that she felt calmer, healthier, and more in control of her mood. Interestingly, she also felt that she was performing better in her job and was more satisfied with her life. She commented that she was surprised at how "slowing down and looking after myself can make so much difference."

Hints and Tips: Overcoming Barriers to Self-Compassion

Often clients do not immediately embrace the idea of self-compassion. Here are some examples of common ways in which clients question the need to take care of themselves, along with some possible answers.

- *"Why should I be kind to myself? Only realistic self-criticism can lead to improvement!"* If this is a client's response to the idea of self-compassion, try to encourage the client to imagine how he or she would relate to a loved one experiencing a similar situation. Would the client be critical to someone who is going through a hard time, or would he or she be supportive and try to make the person feel better and regain confidence, thus increasing the chances of positive future outcomes? Imagining and testing kindness and care toward others can be a way into understanding that it is acceptable to take care of oneself too.

- *"If I sit around indulging myself, I'll never achieve all of things I need or want to do."* Some people with BD set themselves high goals, perhaps unreasonably high. In our experience, traditional verbal challenging of goal striving/high achievement tendencies rarely proves successful. However, an unrelenting push for high goals runs the risk of fueling (hypo) manic symptoms and can also lead to burnout and depression. Metaphors from the sports domain can be helpful here, demonstrating how taking a rest, taking care of the body, and engaging in healthy and "low-key" activities have a positive recovery function—one that does not counteract the aim of achieving further objectives.

- *Other ways of exploring obstacles to self-compassion.* If clients continue to find it difficult to be kind to themselves, despite exploration of these ideas, it can be extremely helpful to use the chair technique mentioned above (and described in detail in Chapter 5) for further exploring any underlying thoughts and assumptions related to self-compassion. These can then be addressed in collaboration with the therapist.

Client Reflection on Being Kind to Oneself

Below is an example of what a MAPP client might say when asked for feedback at the end of treatment, regarding the usefulness of learning about being kind to oneself.

> "Before this therapy, I hadn't realized how strict I always was on myself . . . well, maybe sometimes I did notice it, but I genuinely believed that it was useful, that it would improve things. Talking it through in sessions, I became aware that instead it was a sign of strength to sometimes take time out and look a little bit after myself. it stopped my mood from going lower, which was such a big gain for me!"

CONCLUDING COMMENTS

In this chapter, we have discussed three techniques that we teach all MAPP clients and that form part of the structure of the therapy: how to monitor and cope with fluctuations in mood, and how to be kind to oneself. In the next chapter, we discuss how to approach barriers to successful therapy as they arise.

CHAPTER 5

Overcoming Barriers to Therapy
Chair Work

During the course of psychological therapy, there may be times when both clients and clinicians experience a sense of being "stuck," or feel that a barrier of some kind is impeding progress and preventing necessary work from being done in the therapy sessions. This can occur in all types of psychological therapy, and the MAPP approach is no exception. The question is, how do we overcome these barriers? In MAPP, we have found that a technique called "chair work" can be a useful tool for rapidly "unsticking" difficulties and refocusing on the joint goals of therapy

WHAT IS CHAIR WORK?

Chair work was originally developed as a technique to use in psychodrama (Carstenson, 1955), but it has since been used as an integral part of Gestalt therapy (Perls, 1973) and of schema therapy (Young, Klosko, & Weishaar, 2003).

In the basic version of chair work, two chairs are placed opposite each other. The client sits in one chair and faces the empty chair. The empty chair can represent either a significant other (e.g., a parent, a romantic partner) or a part of the client (e.g., a critical inner voice). The therapist then invites the client to share what the "voice" of the empty chair is saying to him or her. Once this is identified, the therapist can help the client respond to any unhelpful thoughts or beliefs that are blocking progress in therapy by "talking back" to the empty chair.

If it is useful to do so, the client can shuttle back and forth between the two chairs. For example, the client can speak from the part of him- or herself that wants to engage with therapy, and then can switch chairs and speak from the part that is afraid of change.

Additional chairs may be introduced if necessary. This can be useful if the therapist and client are unsure about what might be causing a barrier. Each chair can be used to represent a particular "hypothesis" (generated by either the client or the therapist) about what might be causing the block in therapy, which the therapist can then role-play to see if any of these hypotheses ring true with the client. For example, in a scenario in which there is a chair for the hypothesis that part of the client wants to engage in therapy, and one for the hypothesis that part of the client is afraid of change, there might also be one for the hypothesis that an inner critical voice is "feeding" the fear about engaging in therapy. Further chair work can then take place once the barrier is identified correctly.

In the MAPP approach, the aim of chair work is *only* to overcome barriers in order to allow the client to engage with the imagery-based treatment. The aim of chair work in MAPP is not to work through long-standing relational dynamics or dysfunctional schemas, as might be the case in other therapies.

As this way of working may be unfamiliar to clinicians reading this book, two examples of MAPP chair work are given later in this chapter.

Is It a Useful Approach?

From a CBT perspective, chair work can be a way of "taking what is internal and implicit and making it *external and explicit*" (Goldfried, 1988; emphasis in original). Like other MAPP approaches, chair work is an imagery-based technique, albeit one in which the imaginal component (simulating dialogue with aspects of the self) is aided by physical representations (the chairs). MAPP clients in our case series who used chair work in their sessions often commented that afterward, just imagining the chairs would remind them of important aspects of learning (see the "Client Reflection" at the end of this chapter). Using chairs in this way is a novel experience for most clients, and if the technique is used promptly, it can prevent "stuckness" from setting in over several sessions and becoming entrenched. Certainly it was our experience that the chair work in MAPP was useful and memorable for clients and therapists alike.

Rationale for Chair Work

A therapist might want to explain the rationale for doing chair work in the following way:

"I would be interested to hear your thoughts on this, but I have noticed that we seem to be getting a little 'stuck' in this session. Would you agree?

[Client responds.]

"This is probably going to sound a bit strange, but I suggest we do an exercise now involving chairs. We can use the chairs in the room to represent different ideas, to see whether any seem to resonate or 'fit' with you. Using the chairs can help us to visualize in an external way what might be happening to keep things stuck. You can think of it as another imagery technique, in fact. Once we have a sense of what is going on for you, we might also practice responding to unhelpful ideas by sitting in different chairs and looking at things from different perspectives. How does that sound?"

[In our experience, some clients understand the rationale very easily, while others find the idea of chair work rather peculiar. For those who are unsure, it can be helpful to normalize these feelings of uncertainty and model an experimental, "let's give it a try" approach.]

"We know that what we are suggesting may seem a little unusual, but we can reassure you that previous clients have said that using chairs in this way has been really useful. In fact, these types of chair exercises have been used in therapies for a long time. Would you like to give it a try? We find it's easier to understand it by simply having a go at it. It's normal to be nervous, but we'll guide you through it and support you. What do you say?"

USING CHAIR WORK IN MAPP

In the psychological therapy literature, there are many different permutations of chair work, and indeed one of its advantages is its adaptability. However, in practice, we have tended to use this technique in only two scenarios: (1) when a client's self-criticism is interfering with the progress of therapy, and (2) when it is not clear just what is interfering (and so a client and therapist need to generate hypotheses about the interference).

What follow are detailed examples of how to use chair work in each of these two scenarios. In both these examples, we are assuming that two therapists are present.

Scenario 1: Self-Criticism Interfering with the Intervention

Imagine that a client has done some good imagery work in the previous session with two therapists. However, the client comes to the next session having not practiced the imagery skills at home—something that the client and therapists had jointly agreed would be very useful to do. When the therapists inquire about what made it difficult to practice, the client comments, "I just can't do it. I know it's easy, but I can't get it together to get around to it. I'm useless."

This self-criticism can become noxious if not addressed and can cause a barrier to the client's engaging fully with the imagery work. Therefore, it is worth pausing the therapy at this point and introducing some chair work. One of the therapists can say something like this:

> "It sounds like you are being self-critical, and we've noticed this is something that happens a lot. We are doing some really good work together on your imagery, but then this self-critical voice stops you and makes it really hard for you to do the work. I'd like to suggest that we do a chair exercise to try to understand this more and help you answer back to this voice. It can be a bit unusual, but others have found it helpful. What do you think? Shall we give it a try?"

The therapist takes two chairs and places them facing each other. The client sits in one, and the empty chair represents the self-critical voice. The therapist can sit or stand next to the client, also facing the empty chair. The other therapist can decide whether to sit as an observer or to join the first therapist beside the client.

The first therapist invites the client to repeat what the critical voice says, and, if appropriate, to explore where that voice comes from (though this is not always necessary). Remember, the goal of the exercise is simply to remove the barrier to therapy. The exercise might begin as follows: "Can you repeat what that critical voice is sitting there telling you? Does that remind you of something you have experienced in the past, or a way someone has behaved to you before?"

The next step is to encourage the client to respond to the criticism. If he or she finds it hard, the therapist can model a response in a robust and compassionate way—for example, by saying, "I think what you are saying is really wrong. X is here trying hard; why don't you just leave him [or her] alone? I am really sick of you belittling everything X is trying to do, so just shut up!"

The therapist can then ask the client how the empty chair, representing the other person or the critical voice, would respond. This is important, as a self-critical voice is unlikely to be quieted immediately, and most often a further round of self-criticism will ensue. Again, the therapist asks the client to rebut the criticism, or models how to do this if the client finds it difficult. The client spends a few minutes doing this, and then the cotherapist can physically take the critical chair out of the room. While doing this, the cotherapist might say: "Great! Now I think we should take this chair away completely and lock it out of the room."

This exercise helps the client to identify and externalize an unhelpful critical voice interfering with therapy, and gives him or her the tools to recognize and respond to it. It also gives the therapists an opportunity to model a self-compassionate stance, which the client can then begin to internalize. The banishing of the critical chair is symbolic and memorable.

Exercises such as this can often produce high affect. A supportive, warm, and compassionate stance from the therapists is crucial. Sometimes the client will need strong modeling from the therapists of how to talk to the critical chair.

Scenario 2: Hypothesizing

In the previous scenario, the first therapist identifies quickly that a self-critical voice is interfering with therapy. However, what happens when the therapy just feels "stuck" and no one obvious factor seems to be responsible? This can be frustrating for clients and therapists alike. One of the ways in which we have found chair work particularly helpful in MAPP is to use the chairs as ways of testing hypotheses about what might be responsible for the "stuckness."

Again, imagine that the client and therapists have made good progress with the imagery work in the previous session. At the next session, however, everything stalls, and it seems impossible to pick up the work again. The client says, "I can understand how imagery work might be useful to people, but I just don't think it will work for me. Anyway, the image we worked on last week isn't bothering me." The client then proceeds to talk about a new set of anxieties that the client and therapists have not formulated together.

Does this scenario sound familiar? It can be all too tempting to start working on a new problem instead of continuing with the agreed-upon target. In the MAPP approach, however, we have used chairs to help us collaboratively to think about what might be happening with such a client, so that we can focus on re-engaging with the agreed-upon therapy goal rather than going off in another direction.

In this example, one of the therapists might say something like this:

"Last week we did some really good work together, but today it is feeling like we are struggling to find a way forward. Is that how it feels to you? I'm curious as to what might be going on. I'd like to suggest that we do some more chair work to figure out what is happening here. Is that OK if we try?"

The therapist takes one chair and invites the client to sit in it. The therapist then takes one or more chairs and places them facing the client. Both therapists may well have some ideas or formulations about what is going on, so this is an opportunity for one of them to sit in each "hypothesis" chair in turn and role-play these ideas.

So, for the current scenario, the therapists may hypothesize that today the client is (1) rather depressed and passive; (2) scattered, tangential, and unable to focus; or (3) perhaps dismissive of the intervention. With these ideas in mind, one of the therapists might say something like this:

> "I am not sure what is going on here, but it does feel like we are rather stuck. We have a few hunches about what might be going on, but these are just ideas, so we will need your help. I'm going to sit on these chairs and role-play some different ideas, and you can tell me what you think of them. Does that sound OK to you?"

Then this therapist (or both therapists) can role-play the different hypotheses. For the scenario outlined above, this role play might begin with something like this: "OK, I'm going to make this quite extreme, but remember you are the expert on you. Listen to the ideas, and then let me know what you think."

A therapist sits in the first chair (representing the hypothesis that the client feels depressed and passive) and says, "I've made a mess of lots of things in my life, and I'm no good at working at things. This is just another thing that is not going to work for me, because I'm no good. I'm a hopeless case. I was stupid even to think that this would make a difference to me."

Then a therapist sits in the second chair (representing the hypothesis that the client is feeling scattered and unable to focus) and says,

> "Yes, last week the imagery stuff was good, but everything's changed this week and I have this problem with my roommate, and there's this other really important thing that I should talk to you about too, this weird bubbling I have in my stomach. I haven't thought about the image, but, gosh, I've been having really strange dreams; I wonder if it could be something to do with my diet. Next week I've got so much to do it's all getting on top of me . . ."

Finally, a therapist sits in the last chair (representing the hypothesis that the client is dismissive of the therapy) and says, "I can see how this therapy might work for others, but I am different. I am starting to think that nobody can help me."

The therapists can then ask for feedback from the client about whether any of the hypotheses strikes a chord with him or her. In our experience, clients have a strong "gut" feeling about which process is occurring for them, and often this can be a positive, "aha!" moment for the client that makes sense of why things are feeling stuck. Once a specific barrier is identified, further chair work can be used to respond to the unhelpful "voice" in a way that overcomes the barrier.

Hints and Tips on Using Chair Work

It is common for clinicians unused to this approach to have concerns about using chair work in sessions. An assumption raised frequently is that clients will find the idea stupid or unacceptable in some way and refuse to engage with the technique. In our experience, only rarely do clients respond that way. What we have found useful in allaying clinicians' fears is role-playing chair work scenarios prior to sessions. This is something that can be done easily during supervision (in person or over the telephone) and does not require special training time to be set aside. Chair work needs to be introduced and performed in a curious and collaborative way; it can be framed as clients and therapists trying to work out what is going on. As long as that attitude is present from the start, then there is no pressure on therapists to come up with "solutions" to blocks in therapy; clients and therapists will try to discover the reasons for the blocks together.

CLIENT REFLECTION ON USING CHAIR WORK

The following is a quote from a MAPP client who was asked for feedback at the end of treatment. It reflects the usefulness and power of chair work in dealing with critical inner voices. It also demonstrates that the client was able to use the technique at other times, outside of the therapy.

> "One of my favorite exercises from the MAPP therapy was based on my own impression of having three critical 'voices' following me—positive, neutral, and negative. We took three chairs in the room we were in, and each chair represented one of these voices. As we discussed a situation, I heard the negative voice telling me off. At this point, I literally pushed the chair that was the negative voice out of the room into the corridor—and was quite surprised to hear the voice inside me fading away, once the chair was out of the room. It was a great success! The best part is that once I had done it the first time, it became so easy to imagine kicking that chair out into the corridor any time that voice became too loud and upsetting in my head afterward."

CONCLUDING COMMENTS

Chair work can be an enormously useful tool for rapidly "unsticking" barriers to therapeutic progress. While it might feel a little strange or unfamiliar to start with, clients and therapists alike find it to be memorable and powerful. It can be useful to practice chair work via role play in supervision, to build confidence in using this technique spontaneously when the occasion arises during a therapy session. In fact, role play during supervision in itself can raise insights into why therapy may have become "stuck." We have kept this chapter brief, highlighting the two most frequently occurring scenarios we have used chair work to resolve. However, readers who are eager to know more can consult Arntz and Jacob (2013) for more thorough coverage of the technique and its theoretical background.

PART III
Assessment and Treatment

CHAPTER 6

MAPP Assessment

"Mapping"

In the first stage of MAPP therapy, we offer a detailed, four-session assessment (known as "mapping") to explore or "map out" clients' presenting difficulties. This assessment takes a cognitive-behavioral approach with an imagery focus. The aim of mapping is to identify a target for intervention that is distressing in its own right, but that also has an impact on mood stability. As illustrated in Figure 6.1, we are interested in finding imagery-based phenomena that are distressing a client in the here and now, but that we also hypothesize may have a longer-term impact on the stability of the client's mood (i.e., the extent of the cycling between depression and [hypo]mania).

Importantly, MAPP is not a comprehensive treatment program for BD; instead, it focuses on mapping out and better understanding *one* aspect of bipolar presentation. Once the client's problem is comprehensively mapped out, treatment will then focus on mastering or changing the one aspect. Thus our mapping sessions may differ somewhat from an

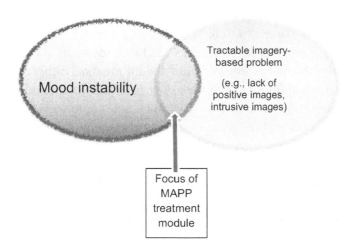

FIGURE 6.1. The MAPP intervention targets—specifically, the intersection between identified, tractable problematic mental imagery (e.g., intrusive negative images or lack of positive imagery) and mood instability.

assessment of BD in traditional CBT. (For example, although we do identify early warning signs of mood episodes with clients, we do not focus on these extensively.)

This chapter is thus a detailed guide on how to conduct a four-session mapping assessment for BD, rather than a guide on how to assess mental imagery in the context of traditional CBT. For further details on how to assess mental imagery generally, see Appendix 1 of this manual, or refer to Hackmann et al. (2011) and Hales et al. (2015).

OVERVIEW OF THE TECHNIQUE

Over the course of the four mapping sessions, areas 1–7 in the list below are assessed and mapped out. These areas are then taken into account when a decision is made on area 8, the selection of a treatment target (or targets).

1. Client's reported priorities.
2. Medication issues.
3. Life chart.
4. Positive coping strategies.
5. Ability to identify prodromes of (hypo)mania and depression.
6. Mapping of imagery/comorbidities influencing mood stability.
7. Initial microformulation of imagery.
8. Selection of treatment target(s).

Later in this chapter, we provide a detailed description of each area of the assessment. Table 6.1 outlines the structure for each of the four mapping sessions. Therapist tasks after each session are also detailed. In MAPP, as in other cognitive-behavioral approaches, our agendas for the session are made explicit. In fact, in MAPP we have a printed agenda for each session, which is placed on a table or in some other convenient location at the start of the session so that the therapist(s) and client can refer to it. This helps to keep the session on track and ensure that the most important items can be covered. These agendas can be found in Appendix 2.

We advise that therapists print out the MAPP Assessment ("Mapping") Document (Appendix 3) and use this document to record the information gathered in these sessions. We have also found it helpful to have a variety of postcards (plain and with pictures) and pens on hand, should clients wish to write their own notes or to record important pieces of learning or strategies to take home with them. (See also Chapter 3 on scaffolding therapy.)

RATIONALE FOR MAPP ASSESSMENT

Below is a suggestion about how to explain the rationale for MAPP assessment or "mapping" to a client:

"Welcome to today's session. As you know, this is the first of four 'mapping' sessions that we will meet for. As the name 'mapping' suggests, in these first four sessions we will

TABLE 6.1. What to Cover in Each of the Four MAPP Assessment ("Mapping") Sessions

<u>Session 1</u>

- Client and therapist(s) introduce themselves.
- Set agenda.
- Introduce mapping model (structure, client requirements, end criteria).
- Describe aim and purpose of mapping.
- Begin mapping, using the MAPP Assessment ("Mapping") Document (Appendix 3) to record details.

- *Main tasks for session 1:*
  - Confirm reason for referral.
  - Review client's current mood (using scores on standardized questionnaires such as the QIDS, ASRM, and BAI, completed prior to or in the session)
  - Ascertain client's reported priorities (cross-check with referral letter).
  - Discuss any medication issues.
  - Start assessment of imagery/comorbidities influencing mood stability.
  - Start recording of current positive coping strategies.

- Check that future mapping sessions are scheduled.

- *Therapist postsession tasks:*
  - Record notes in line with service's or health care provider's guidelines.
  - Begin to write mapping report.

<u>Session 2</u>

- Client and therapist(s) greet each other (or introduce themselves, if one therapist has not yet met the client).
- Set agenda.
- Review client's mood (as above).
- Review information covered in mapping session 1.
- Continue mapping, using the MAPP Assessment ("Mapping") Document (Appendix 3).

- *Main tasks for session 2:*
  - Begin life chart. Record periods of anxiety, depression, and (hypo)mania above the line, and life events below the line.
  - Assess client's ability to identify early warning signs of (hypo)mania and depression.
  - Continue investigation of imagery/comorbidities influencing mood stability.
  - Begin microformulation of imagery (if possible).
  - Add information to other sections in mapping report if it arises.

- If appropriate, therapist(s) can select specific standardized questionnaires for client to fill in, based on information gained in mapping (e.g., to assess social anxiety).
- Therapist(s) and client agree on individualized visual analogue scales to rate clinically important aspects of identified imagery.
- Assign homework: Client to continue working on life chart (if appropriate).
- Photocopy life chart for client to take home and work on if he or she wishes.

- *Therapist postsession tasks:*
  - Record notes in line with service's or health care provider's guidelines.
  - Continue to write mapping report; have draft ready to discuss in the next session.

<u>Session 3</u>

- Client and therapist(s) greet each other (or introduce themselves, if one therapist has not yet met the client).
- Set agenda.

(continued)

TABLE 6.1. *(continued)*

- Review client's mood (briefly).
- Review homework of completing life chart (if this was assigned); add further information.
- Review draft of mapping report.
- Therapist(s) to feed back to client whether a MAPP treatment module is indicated.

- *Main tasks for session 3:*
  - Client and therapist(s) jointly amend mapping report.
  - Refine microformulation of imagery, with aim of identifying concrete intervention targets.
  - Flesh out other sections of report if necessary.
  - Include any further information in report that therapist(s) or client perceives as useful. (The mapping report is to be viewed as a document that provides a useful summary of information for the client and for other professionals who may be involved in the client's care.)

- *Therapist postsession tasks:*
  - Record notes in line with service's or health care provider's guidelines.
  - Amend mapping report to include client feedback.

Session 4

- Client and therapist(s) greet each other (or introduce themselves, if one therapist has not yet met the client).
- Set agenda.
- Review client's mood (briefly).
- Review revised mapping report.

- *Main tasks for session 4:*
  - Agree on MAPP treatment module target (if treatment module is offered).
  - Seek client's feedback on his or her experience of mapping—what was useful/not useful.
  - Explain MAPP treatment procedure.

- Confirm dates for MAPP treatment module.

- *Therapist postsession tasks:*
  - Record notes in line with service's or health care provider's guidelines.
  - Send final mapping report to referring clinician and copied to client, client's health care provider, and any other health care professionals that the client would like to receive a copy.

Note. Adapted from Hales et al. (2015). Copyright © 2015 by The Guilford Press. Adapted by permission.

focus on understanding what difficulties you are currently having, and will try to identify and map out what types of things have an impact on your mood stability, particularly relating to mental imagery and anxiety. At the end of these four sessions, we may have decided on a specific target to work on in your treatment sessions. Alternatively, we may decide that the mapping exercise has been sufficiently useful on its own and that no further treatment is necessary. Does that make sense?

"There are a few things about MAPP that may differ from psychology appointments you've had before. [When cotherapists are present:] First, you will have noticed that there are two therapists here. This is because, in our experience, we find that it's really helpful to be able to put three heads together rather than just two, to think about things in different ways and from different viewpoints. Our clients have said that although they might find this a little unusual at first, it is something that they tend to get used to quickly and really value.

"The second thing [when cotherapists are present]/The main thing [when one therapist is present] is that the MAPP approach is quite brief and structured, which may be different from what you are used to. We think that it's most helpful to focus on a specific difficulty—one that has an impact on your mood stability. First we will map it out to understand it, and then we will really make sure we focus on that one difficulty in treatment, to get to the bottom of it. What we aim to do in our mapping sessions is find out what might be the most useful focus of treatment for you as an individual. In MAPP, we don't try to treat every part of bipolar disorder that might be a difficulty. We prioritize one 'piece of the puzzle' and work on providing a really good treatment for this specific 'piece.' This means that we may at times decide to put aside other issues that crop up, in the interests of holding to our agreed-upon focus. Do you have any questions about that?"

GETTING INFORMATION ABOUT EACH AREA TO BE ASSESSED

Below, we describe each area to be assessed in the "mapping" sessions in further detail.

Area 1: Client's Reported Priorities

In the first session, one of the key aims is to gain an understanding of what the client thinks are his or her main difficulties and priorities to address in treatment. The aim at this stage of mapping is broadly to elicit the client's current concerns, rather than to undertake a detailed exploration of each priority.

Clients may report priorities that are quite general, such as "to increase my self-worth," or may state specific targets they would like to work on, such as "to reduce my anxiety in social performance situations." Both of these types of priorities are valid. We would suggest, however, that a maximum of three priorities per client be chosen for discussion and brief exploration. Here are some examples of priorities reported by previous clients:

- To reduce intrusive traumatic/distressing imagery from the past.
- To find ways of coping with distressing images of the future.
- To address perceptual distortion in the here and now (e.g., seeing people from an observer's perspective).
- To address anxiety and negative imagery related to insecurity about current relationships.
- To find strategies to stabilize energy levels.
- To address intrusive negative imagery leading to angry feelings/outbursts toward others.

Sometimes a client may report that he or she wants to work on something that may not be possible to do in a brief, focused treatment approach. For example, the client may say that a priority is "to understand why I keep behaving in the same way over and over again in my romantic relationships." In such cases, the therapist(s) may gently remind the client of the brief nature of the intervention and inquire whether there is something more specific within this broad concern that the client thinks he or she could work on. Socratic questions may reveal, for example, that the client's behavior is linked to social anxiety or negative self-imagery (which then could form a useful treatment target within this broader goal).

Area 2: Medication Issues

In MAPP, we recognize that effective treatment of BD often warrants a joint psychological and pharmacotherapeutic approach (see Chapter 3 on the MAPP therapeutic ethos).

In this part of the mapping procedure, a therapist asks whether a client is currently taking medication; if so, whether there are any difficulties with medication compliance (e.g., unwillingness to take medications because of side effects); and whether there are any further medication issues of note (e.g., concerns about taking medications and wanting to start a family). From the outset, it is made clear that this information will be communicated to psychiatric colleagues in a transparent way, particularly findings related to issues of medication compliance (e.g., a client reports discontinuing medication) and risk.

Area 3: Life Chart

The life chart area of the mapping procedure takes the form of a timeline (it may be as simple as a horizontal line drawn on a landscape piece of paper), which is collaboratively filled in by the client and therapist(s). The left end of the line represents the date the client was born; the right end represents the present day. In the top section of the paper, above the line, the client maps episodes of mood disturbance or anxiety. In the bottom section of the paper, below the line, the client maps important life events (which can be positive, negative, or neutral). See Figure 6.2 for an example of a life chart.

If information is already known about a client's history before the mapping sessions begin, then a therapist can add this information to the timeline in advance of the session (e.g., major mood episodes, hospitalizations, significant life events) if the client feels that this is useful.

The life chart is started in session 2. The client can continue to work on the timeline between sessions if he or she desires. If so, the timeline should be photocopied, and the client should be given the copy. However, working on the timeline between sessions is not mandatory. Some clients may prefer the therapist(s) to keep the timeline for them, particularly if difficult events or times have been discussed.

The life chart exercise can help identify patterns in triggers for mood episodes—for example, that hypomania typically follows life transitions such as moving to a new house or changing jobs. It can also highlight times of stability and factors influencing stable mood. Our clients report that this exercise is useful to them and helps build a coherent sense of the link between life events and mood.

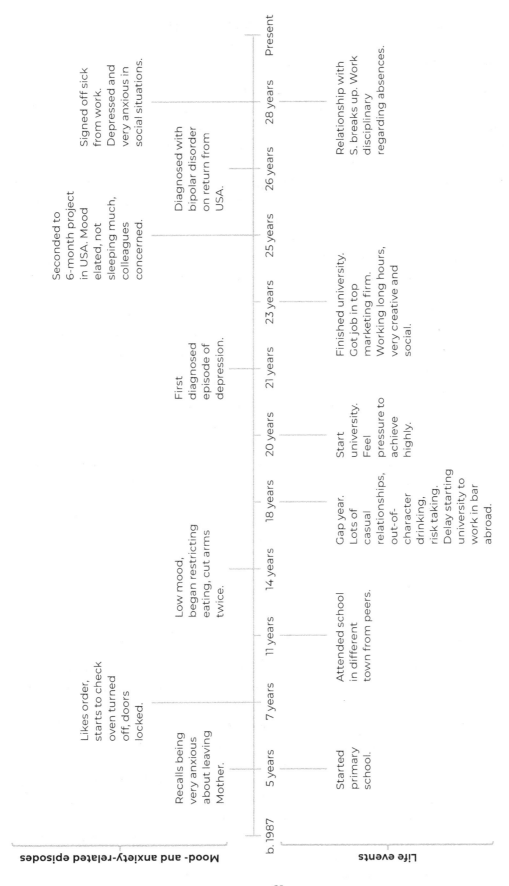

FIGURE 6.2. Example of a client's life chart. (Clarification of U.K. idioms for U.S. readers: "Seconded to 6-month project" means "Assigned to . . ."; "Signed off sick from work" means "Took extended period of sick leave"; "Work disciplinary" means "Disciplined at work.")

61

Area 4: Positive Coping Strategies

Information for the section on positive coping strategies can be collected in two ways. First, therapists can directly ask clients whether they currently use any strategies (e.g., talking about anxieties with others, exercising, limiting activities when overly energetic) that have a positive impact on their mood stability, or have helped to reduce symptoms of (hypo)mania/depression/anxiety in the past.

However, while clients may be able to report on some strategies that they use consciously, there may also be less explicitly known strategies that therapists can help the clients to identify over the course of the mapping.

For example, while completing the life chart, one client noticed that his periods of depression tended to coincide with times when he was living alone and having reduced social contact. Through discussion with his therapists, he realized that one positive strategy he currently used when feeling low was to say yes to social invitations, even if he did not feel like keeping these engagements at the time. He generally found that he enjoyed these occasions even when he did not expect to, which had a corresponding positive impact on his mood. The client and therapists concluded that maintaining regular social contact with others, especially in times of low mood, was a positive coping strategy; they subsequently recorded it in this section of the report. Therapists should therefore remain alert to positive coping strategies implied or stated by clients throughout the course of the whole mapping procedure, and record these in this section.

It is worth noting that clients often underestimate the impact of behavioral factors such as disrupted sleep–wake routines, poor diet, use of alcohol/other substances, limited exercise, and so forth on their moods. So we advocate including positive behavioral strategies in this section, as well as cognitive/social strategies. These types of strategies are used widely in other successful psychoeducational and behavioral approaches to managing BD (e.g., see Frank, 2005; Lam, Jones, & Hayward, 2010). Such strategies may be as simple as "getting up and going to bed at the same time every day," "not drinking more than one glass of wine per day," and so on.

Area 5: Ability to Identify Prodromes of (Hypo)mania and Depression

"Prodromes," or "early warning signs" (EWS), are changes and symptoms that may herald the onset of a relapse of (hypo)mania or depression. As mentioned earlier, MAPP, unlike pure psychoeducational approaches, does not focus *extensively* on identification of EWS of mood episodes. However, this is considered a useful section of mapping, and time should be allocated to it. (For further information on psychoeducational approaches to BD, see Colom & Lam, 2005; Colom & Vieta, 2006; Miklowitz et al., 2012.)

In this part of the assessment, therapists think with clients about whether they can identify their individual EWS, and then specifically record any elicited EWS for episodes of depression, (hypo)mania, and (if anxiety is comorbid) anxiety.

As there are for identifying positive coping strategies, there are two ways of identifying EWS. The first is to directly ask clients what, if anything, they notice when they are beginning to feel depressed, overly elated, or anxious. Clients can sometimes clearly articulate particular indicators that they use to gauge a shift in mood, and these should therefore be recorded. If clients are less able to identify EWS, then therapists can use a variety of Socratic techniques to help them think about their prodromal periods and prompt them to identify EWS.

For example, a client and therapist(s) can review the client's mood chart collaboratively and identify a point where a mood shift began to occur. Holding this period in mind, the client can then be asked to try to recall any particular symptoms (e.g., sleeping more or less, a sense of lethargy/energy) or changes in behavior (e.g., withdrawing from others, unusual overspending) that may have begun at this point.

It is common for clients to report that they are less able to spot the EWS of (hypo) mania, which often means that they are less likely to put in place coping strategies to stabilize elevating mood. It can therefore often be particularly helpful to think about EWS in this domain.

Area 6: Assessment of Imagery/Comorbidities Influencing Mood Stability

It is helpful for therapists to keep the model illustrated in Figure 6.1 in mind when completing this section of the assessment. The aim is to identify and formulate potential tractable targets for treatment. By "tractable," we mean something that (1) is having an impact on a client's mood stability and (2) can feasibly be addressed *within the time-limited MAPP treatment module.*

Therapists can use clients' priorities as a starting point for exploration of the potential impact of imagery or comorbidities on their mood stability. For example, the following exchange might take place:

THERAPIST: You told me the thing that you find most difficult at the moment is coping with depression. Have I understood that correctly?

CLIENT: Yes.

THERAPIST: Can you tell me the last time you felt very down? Was it this week?

CLIENT: Yes.

THERAPIST: Can you tell me what you were doing at that time?

CLIENT: I had been trying to finish an essay that was due the next day, and I just felt like I couldn't do it and that what I had written was a piece of crap, and I just felt awful.

THERAPIST: And when you were trying to finish the essay and you were feeling awful, did any images or thoughts come to mind?

CLIENT: Ummm, yes, actually, I did . . . uh, this is going to sound really weird, but I was thinking about how I was going to fail my course and not get a job and I'd end up kind of . . . um . . . just kind of mentally ill and raggedy and on the streets.

THERAPIST: And did you see that image of yourself in the future in your mind's eye?

CLIENT: Yes, yes, I did.

THERAPIST: And what impact did that have on your mood?

CLIENT: Not a good one! It made me feel really bad, like there was no point in trying any more.

THERAPIST: Did any other images come with it?

CLIENT: Yes . . . (*Voice trails off, and client looks sad and uncomfortable.*)

THERAPIST: Sometimes when people feel very low, they can experience images of harming themselves. Were those types of images in mind?

CLIENT: I get them quite a lot. They scare me, and I haven't really spoken about them to anyone.

THERAPIST: I understand that they must be scary. Can you describe what you see?

CLIENT: I see myself hanging. There's this tree I pass on my way to the shops, and I can't stop imagining myself . . .

THERAPIST: When you have that image of yourself hanging, what impact does it have on you?

CLIENT: Well, it makes me feel scared, because I think, "Well, I might do this. I might not be able to stop myself."

THERAPIST: And then what does it make you want to do?

CLIENT: Just hide myself away really, stop going out, avoid going past the tree . . .

The exchange above highlights the impact of imagery on the client's mood state and suggests that further exploration is warranted (i.e., that this image could be a reasonable treatment target). We don't assume that all images will have a significant impact on mood stability. Rather, we look for those images that lead to clear feelings of distress (such as anxiety) and that, on further exploration, we find do have a longer-lasting impact on mood.

Also, more than one image or type of image can be identified; clients may report different types of imagery in different mood states. For example, a client may report energizing, positive imagery in manic states, as opposed to imagery of a hopeless future in depressed states (as illustrated above).

If clients are struggling to describe any mental imagery, it can be helpful to have them fill in some standardized imagery measures (indeed, this can be helpful for clinicians anyway) as a way of cueing them in to mental imagery experiences. In MAPP, we routinely use two imagery measures to aid our understanding of clients' experiences: the Spontaneous Use of Imagery Scale (SUIS; Reisberg, Pearson, & Kosslyn, 2003), a measure of general use of imagery in everyday life; and the Impact of Future Events Scale (IFES; Deeprose & Holmes, 2010), a measure of intrusive future-oriented imagery.

Area 7: Initial Microformulation of Imagery

Once an image has been identified that has a plausible link with the client's mood stability, an initial microformulation can be collaboratively developed with the client. Detailed instructions for how to complete the microformulation are provided in Chapter 7.

Note that only a rough microformulation is needed at this point—enough to be able to fill in the Microformulation Template (Appendix 4). If the image is chosen as a treatment target, there will be time to expand the microformulation and deepen understanding of the image during the treatment phase.

Area 8: Selection of Treatment Target(s)

In the final assessment session, a treatment target (or targets, but usually just one) for the intervention part of the MAPP procedure should be chosen. The client and therapists will collaboratively decide on a treatment target, based on the information gained in the mapping. It is expected that the treatment target will be one that has been microformulated (i.e., a new topic is not normally chosen in session 4); has a plausible link with the client's mood stability; is deemed to be tractable; and is suitable for a brief intervention (i.e., not one that relates to long-term relational dynamics or dysfunctional schemas).

A question that frequently arises when we are describing the MAPP approach to clinicians is this: "But how do you know which image to work with?" From the mapping assessment, it should be clear whether the client:

1. Has a recurrent single image (or small set of images) linked to mood stability (i.e., tending to escalate low, high, or anxious mood).
2. Experiences a plethora of images that change from day to day but nonetheless have a large impact on mood stability.
3. Has a paucity of positive images to draw upon.

Different imagery techniques are better suited to each of these three options. Thus it is helpful to think about which imagery techniques might best address the mapped images at assessment, and then to use this as a guide for decision making.

The aims of different imagery techniques used in MAPP are outlined below (see Chapter 7 for a more detailed list of which techniques to consider for each kind of microformulation).

• *Metacognitive strategies.* The aim of these strategies is to reduce the power of an image by changing how a client relates to it. They do not target the content of an image. In essence, their aim is to change how the client responds to an image—by shifting attention away from it, or by doing something that reinforces that it is just an image and not "real." Metacognitive techniques can be especially useful when a client describes being besieged by images of many different types, as in option 2 in the list just above.

• *Imagery rescripting.* This technique can be used with images of actual events (memories), or of imagined past, current, or future events. The overall aim is to change how the image makes the client feel. Imagery rescripting tends to work best when a single image (or small set of images) is identified by the client as problematic, as in option 1 in the list above.

• *Positive imagery.* The third set of strategies involves creating new stand-alone positive imagery. We tend to use a free-standing positive image when there are too many images to rescript individually (as in option 2 above), or where the client needs help to increase his or her ability to self-soothe (as in option 3 above).

  • *Imagery-competing tasks.* These final techniques can be useful when a client is unable to engage in imagery rescripting—for example, if the image is too distressing, if an immediate coping strategy is needed, or if there are just too many images to work on (as in option 2 above).

Considering these four kinds of imagery techniques should guide clinicians toward deciding which of the problematic images identified at assessment to pick as the treatment target(s).

CASE EXAMPLE: EVAN

Evan was a mechanic in his late 30s who had recently been divorced. He had a teenage son who, since the separation, he saw only on weekends. Evan had been diagnosed with BD in his early 20s, following a period of what he described as "very wild behavior." Since his diagnosis, he had generally managed his BD well by using a combination of medication and behavioral strategies, such as cutting out alcohol and maintaining a steady schedule. However, in the month preceding our first meeting, relatives had expressed concerns that Evan was uncharacteristically "low" and irritable. This had prompted his psychiatrist to make a referral to MAPP.

When we first met with Evan, he was depressed and rather reserved. He reported that he was working long hours as a way of getting through the week, and had stopped seeing friends with whom he usually played sports. He said that he had initially coped well with his divorce, as it was mutually agreed upon, but that he was now finding being apart from his son very tough and was worried about how the boy was coping at school.

When we explored Evan's feelings about his relationship with his son in more detail, we discovered that he was experiencing a strong intrusive image of himself as an old, ill man, sitting on a park bench alone. He was very tearful as he described the image and said, "I feel I have lost him [my son] and I will always be alone." Understandably, this image made him feel very hopeless and depressed. It was particularly sad that the image had led him to emotionally withdraw a little from his son during the time they did have together.

We also discussed Evan's concerns about his son's experience at school, and he reported repeatedly imagining him getting into fights at school, without Evan there to protect him. This would make him feel both angry and impotent as a father. However, on further exploration, Evan was also able to identify that there was no evidence that his son was getting into fights; rather, he was instead imagining the worst-case scenario, just as he had been with the image of himself alone on a bench in the park.

Evan reported that before the MAPP assessment, he had not seen the future scenarios he was automatically imagining as "just mental images," but had considered them certainties of his life to come. Being able to step back from the images and understand the power they were wielding over him made him hopeful that he might be able to change things and influence his future for the better. He was offered a treatment module to target his problematic imagery, focused on first changing his relationship with mental imagery via metacognitive techniques, and then using imagery rescripting to target specific distressing images of the future.

CLIENT REFLECTION ON MAPP ASSESSMENT

The following is a quote from a MAPP client who was asked for feedback at the end of treatment. It reflects the usefulness of a thorough assessment.

"When they told me that they would spend four whole sessions mapping out my difficulties, I thought we would be twiddling our thumbs . . . but it was surprising how much there was to understand and how different things were interrelated. I liked the detail we went into about my images—it really made sense by the end. I've seen lots of different people over the years, but none of them have ever stayed on one thing until we really got to the bottom of it before—brilliant!"

CONCLUDING COMMENTS

In this chapter, we have discussed how to assess or "map out" clients' difficulties over four sessions. Although this might seem like quite a lot of time to spend on assessment, a thorough understanding of how mental imagery interacts with the rest of a client's life is important for selecting the correct treatment target(s). In the next chapter, we explain more about how to microformulate an image; we then discuss providing clients with psychoeducation about some of the scientific research that explains why mental images can have such a profound impact on emotion.

CHAPTER 7

Microformulation of a Particular Mental Image, and Psychoeducation for Clients

This chapter covers the two important components of the MAPP protocol that precede treatment. First, we describe how to explore and understand a particular mental image—a process we call "microformulation." Next, we outline the psychoeducational material about mental imagery that it is helpful to share with clients.

MICROFORMULATION OF AN IMAGE

To review the discussion of imagery in earlier chapters, while we tend to think of something visual when we talk about images, a mental image can involve any of the senses: vision, hearing, smell, taste, and/or touch.

Exploration of a particular mental image tends to occur in two main places within MAPP therapy. First, a brief/rough microformulation may occur in the context of going through the client's priorities for treatment, trying to select a treatment target. Second, once the client and therapist(s) have selected an image to work on and are in the treatment phase, a more detailed microformulation is needed. In both cases, the aim is to be in a position to fill out (in varying degrees of detail) the Microformulation Template (Appendix 4; see Figures 8.1, 9.7, 10.2, and 11.1 for filled-in examples of a modified Microformulation Template for four different clients).

"Microformulation" (Hackmann et al., 2011) is a process similar to developing a typical collaborative CBT case formulation. However, it differs from standard CBT case conceptualization in that the presenting difficulty (the troublesome mental imagery) is not put at the center of a comprehensive case formulation—that is, one taking into account the client's entire social, familial, and psychiatric history (although this may happen at a later stage). Rather, the focus is on the image in its own right; its content and effects are mapped out in detail. This microformulation will deepen everyone's understanding of the image: what it is, why it persists, and how it affects the client's mood. In addition, it will begin to show the therapist(s) how and where intervention may be possible.

Rationale for Microformulation

To introduce microformulation to a client, a therapist might want to say something like this:

> "Today we would like to focus on one image. This might be the one you most want to work on, or the one that most troubles you, or one that we think would make a huge difference if we were able to change it a bit. We are going to try to map out the impact it has on you. When we have done that, we might be able to look at various things we can try, so that it doesn't keep going around and around in your head, and coming back again and again."

Description of Steps

There are seven steps in microformulation:

1. Choose an image to microformulate.
2. Ask the client for a rich description of the image.
3. Identify the emotions in the image.
4. Identify the appraisals in the image.
5. Identify the power of the image (i.e., do a metacognitive appraisal of the image—why it is not dismissed or ignored, why it matters).
6. Identify the responses that maintain the image.
7. Identify the triggers and original source (if relevant) of the image.

We explain each step in detail below. The completion of the microformulation should be a collaborative, curiosity-driven process, with responsibility for completion shared equally between the therapist(s) and the client. We do not want the therapist(s) to be doing something to or for the client; we want them to uncover information and gain insight together. With this in mind, it is a good idea in session to place a blank copy of the Microformulation Template where it can be seen by both the therapist(s) and the client, such as on a table between them. In addition, encourage the client to write on the template him- or herself, unless the client really does not wish to do so.

Step 1: Choose an Image to Microformulate

Any client may report more than one significant image. When a client and therapist(s) are deciding which one to pick to start microformulation, it might be useful to consider these questions:

- Is there an image that the client is most interested in working with, or one that is most significant to him or her?
- Is there an image that seems directly connected to the treatment target identified by the client?
- Is there an image that is relevant to the client's current clinical presentation and has been present in the week(s) preceding the session?
- Is there an image that the therapist(s) think might be tractable (i.e., that is likely to respond to mental imagery techniques) in a short number of sessions?

Below are some useful questions to ask to assess for the presence and possible impact of imagery on mood stability:

"When you are feeling depressed [anxious, high, etc.], is there a common or repeated image that comes to mind?"

"Does your mental imagery change depending on how you are feeling? For example, do you notice that you experience different types of mental imagery when you are depressed compared to when you are anxious [high, etc.]?"

"Which image do you feel is most significant for you? How frequently do you experience this image?"

"If you bring this image to mind now, how does it make you feel?"

"Does the imagery have any meanings associated with it—for example, how you think about yourself or others?"

"When you have the image, how much do you believe the meanings in the image?"

"Does the imagery make you want to do anything in response to it? How compelling is the imagery?"

Step 2: Ask the Client for a Rich Description of the Image

Once an image has been chosen, the client is asked to provide a description of the image that is so full and detailed that therapists can see it (or hear it, taste it, etc.) themselves. If they can't, they need to ask the client for more details. This process can start with asking the client to remember the last time he or she had the image, and then to bring it back to mind and describe it in as much detail as possible. (Having the client keep his or her eyes closed for this is preferable, but is not completely necessary.)

To introduce this step to the client, a therapist might want to say something like this:

"Now I know you have told me a bit about the image, but the next step is for you to give me a really detailed description of it. I am going to ask you all about what you can see, hear, smell, taste, feel . . . whatever, all of the details. Also, about what happens in the image and when. This is because I want to be able to understand it well enough to see it myself, inside my own head. Is that OK?

[Client responds.]

"So when was the last time that you had that image?

[Client responds.]

"OK, can I get you to close your eyes and take yourself back to that moment? What were you doing? Where were you?

[Client responds.]

"OK, now can you get the image back in your head? Is it there? Now can you describe it to me in the first person and the present tense—that is, 'I can see X and I can hear Y'?"

Therapists should try to find out:

- How the image would look if the therapists could see it themselves.
- From which perspective the image is seen. In other words, is the client in the picture, viewing him- or herself from outside (i.e., the "observer" perspective), or is the client viewing the scene through his or her own eyes (i.e., the "field" perspective)?
- Whether the image is still like a photograph or moving like a film.
- All the details about dimensions and colors.
- If and how the image changes (elements/people coming and going).
- If there is any action going on, and whether the client is involved in it.
- What the client can hear, smell, taste, and feel physically in the image.

Every few sentences, a therapist should summarize back to the client what the client has said so far about the image. This will serve two useful purposes: It will act as a check that the therapists have understood the client correctly, and it will prompt him or her to remember more details. For example, a therapist might say something like this:

"OK, so far you have told me you see a picture of yourself running down a country lane in the dark. You are viewing the image through your own eyes. It is cold, and you can feel the wind on your skin. You are wearing a white cotton nightdress, which feels a little damp against your skin. You can hear the rustling of animals in the undergrowth beside you and the sound of your own breathing, panting. Your chest feels tight, and your legs ache. Do I have it right so far? What have I missed?

[Client responds.]

"Can you smell anything in the image or taste anything in your mouth?"

Occasionally, clients find it hard to give a rich description of an image. This may be because they find the image too threatening to dwell on. If this is the case, it might be worth starting with an image that is a little less "hot." However, if clients have trouble describing an image because they are not used to describing things in such a detailed way, then it is worth having them practice describing more neutral mental images first. This could begin with getting such clients to close their eyes and undertake an imaginary walk around their apartment, flat, or house. A therapist can guide such a client as follows:

"Start at the front door (describe it, its color, the sounds you hear, the smells . . .)."

"Take out your key and open the door (feel the key, feel the movement, any sound . . .)."

"Walk into the first room (describe the temperature, what you can see, hear, smell . . .)."

"Bend down and take off your shoes and wiggle your toes (describe it, feel the movement, feel the floor against your bare feet . . .)."

"Walk to the kitchen and open the fridge (describe it, the sound, the temperature . . .)."

"Take out some food, such as a lemon (describe it, feel the movement, the temperature . . .)."

"Taste the food (describe the taste/texture/smell . . .)."

Now have the client simply continue with any other rooms, moving around within them and describing them, until he or she seems to have the idea.

Once the client has learned how to describe this neutral image in detail, he or she should be able to transfer the skill to more troubling images.

Step 3: Identify the Emotions in the Image

In the third step, the client and therapist(s) identify the emotion or emotions in the image—how the image makes the client *feel*. In MAPP, this is the most important part of an image, and the thing that the treatment will aim to change later. We know that images influence emotions more than verbal thoughts do, so the emotions carried by an image are likely to be potent.

A therapist needs simply to ask the client how the client feels as he or she holds the image in mind, or how the client felt on the last occasion he or she experienced it. If this is difficult for the client to do, the therapist(s) should observe the client's body language as he or she is imagining. This may provide some clues about the emotions the client is experiencing. A therapist can suggest the feelings he or she is inferring to the client and see whether the client agrees. Alternatively, a therapist can read out the description of the image from step 2 and ask the client how specific details and features in the image make him or her feel.

An image can elicit more than one emotion; the therapist(s) should write down as many emotions as are present. Sometimes clients will not use standard labels to describe emotions, but will use more metaphorical attributes. It is OK to keep the client's exact words in this case, provided that the client is asked to explain fully what he or she means, so that the therapist(s) can share the "felt sense" behind each word.

A therapist might want to introduce this step as follows:

"Can I ask you to bring the image you have just described back into your mind? Can you see it clearly?

[Client responds.]

"Would it help if I described it back to you again? Now hold it in your mind and tell me how it makes you feel. What emotions do you experience when it is in your mind?

[Client responds.]

"So when this image is in your mind, you feel *X*. What other emotions do you feel?" [This question is repeated until there are no more emotions. It might help to give examples of a range of emotions.]

Step 4: Identify the Appraisals in the Image

In the fourth step, the client and therapist(s) need to find out what is generating the emotions identified in step 3. What is the client thinking that is leading him or her to feel *X, Y, Z*? The way to find this out is by asking the client why he or she feels the various emotions just described or what thoughts run through his or her mind as the client holds the image in mind. Obviously, if many emotions are evoked by the image, then the appraisals that lie behind each one will need to be identified. In addition, several slightly different appraisals may be generating the same emotion, so it is worth checking that there isn't more than one appraisal per emotion.

A therapist might want to introduce this step as follows:

"While you still have the image in your mind, can we focus on the part where you feel [for example] scared? Do you have that in mind now? Why do you think you are feeling scared? What is running through your mind that is making you feel scared? What are you scared about/scared of?

[Client responds.]

"OK, so you are thinking [for example], 'My daughter is going to get seriously ill,' and that is making you feel scared. Is that right? Is there anything else that you are thinking that is making you feel scared?

[Client responds.]

"Can we move on to the part where you feel [for example] sad? Do you have that in mind now? Why do you think you are feeling sad?" [The questioning continues as before.]

For this part of the microformulation, it is worth taking some time and being a little bit "forensic" about the appraisals being gathered. The eventual aim of producing a microformulation is to change the image and/or its meaning so that it is not generating unhelpful and mood-destabilizing emotions. Understanding the meaning behind the emotions correctly is therefore *crucial*. It might help to produce a chart listing all of the emotions and their associated meanings, as shown in the example in Figure 7.1. (A blank version of this chart is available as Appendix 5.)

This chart should be placed so that everyone can see it. Together, the client and therapist(s) should check that the appraisals "match" the emotions (i.e., that those appraisals really are what the client is thinking that makes him or her feel the given emotions). A useful tip is to apply the "1,000 people test": Would all of a group of 1,000 people, on thinking the thought (and believing it), feel that same emotion? If the answer is no, it may be

For the target image, fill in the emotion(s) that you feel while you hold it in mind. Then, establish what you are thinking/what is running through your mind that is making you feel that emotion. Ensure that you establish this information for *all* of the emotions that you feel when you hold the image in mind.

Image	Emotions: How do you feel?	Appraisals: When you feel X, what is running through your mind? What are you thinking that is making you feel X?
Image of daughter	Scared	She is going to get seriously ill.
	Sad	She will die.

FIGURE 7.1. Example of a filled-in Chart for Recording Emotions and Appraisals within a Troublesome Image (Appendix 5).

that there is another thought that hasn't been uncovered yet. A good example would be the client's appraisal from the example just above that "My daughter is going to get seriously ill." While many people *would* feel sad on thinking and believing that thought, it does not pass the 1,000 people test. Some people would feel scared only, or scared but hopeful that everything might be OK in the end; sadness implies a definite bad ending. Further questioning about what lies behind the sadness might then uncover the true appraisal—that the daughter will die. Feeling sad at the idea of one's daughter dying *would* pass the 1,000 people test.

Step 5: Identify the Power of the Image

In the fifth step, the client and therapist(s) want to discover why the client is unable or unwilling to ignore or dismiss the image. They are attempting to answer this question: What are the good reasons why this client does not just think, "It's only an image; it doesn't mean anything; it's just inside my head"? In other words, this step involves searching for a more metacognitive element to the microformulation. Because of the multisensory, vivid nature of imagery, people often misinterpret an image as being a reflection of reality. Moreover, as we discuss later in this chapter, scientific research into mental imagery shows us that people's brains are often reacting to images as if they reflect reality. This mental process is automatic, and therefore people often automatically respond as if the image is real too. In this step, therapists are trying to draw the client's and their own attention to this automatic process and response.

Once the main emotions and the appraisals linked to the emotions have been identified, useful questions to investigate the power of the image include the following:

> "When you have that experience, does it feel real, like something actually happening in the outside world? Or do you just see it and realize it's just a thought in your head? What is it about the image that makes it feel so real?"

> "Does it feel like something happening now?"

> "Does it seem like a premonition?"

> "Are you afraid you might go mad, die, collapse, or be overwhelmed if you allow this image into your mind?"

> "Do you think it could affect other people?"

> "Do you think that holding that image in mind could suck you back into the past/into another reality?"

> "What does it mean to you that you have this image?"

In our experience, often the clue to uncovering the power of an image lies in the sense a client makes of its vividness. Because images can be so absorbing and have such a great impact on emotions, clients comment that they "feel so real" that they think the images must be true or prophetic in some way. Thus the power-of-the-image part of the microformulation often starts with this sentence: "The image is so vivid that . . ." Alternatively, because images have such an impact on emotions, clients can think that they may damage themselves or others if they continue to experience these images.

Occasionally, clients may be embarrassed to admit that they believe an image may be prophetic or may represent reality. Having a printed list of possible reasons behind the power of the image, which the therapist(s) can explain have been gathered from other clients, might have a normalizing effect.

Reasons Clients Often Give to Explain Why They Cannot Ignore or Dismiss an Image

"It is very vivid, so it must be true/real."

"I can hear/smell/feel it, so it must be true."

"It is so clear and bright and strong, it must mean something/it must be a warning."

"It is so vivid, it must be prophetic/it must be going to come true."

"It is so strong and upsetting that I think that if I dwell on it, it will make me go mad/ collapse/be overwhelmed. . . . I won't be able to cope."

"It is so powerful that I fear it may harm me/others."

"It is so clear and real . . . I can smell it/taste it/hear it/feel it on my skin . . . it feels as if it is happening now."

"It is so strong and happens so much, it must mean that I want it to happen."

Step 6: Identify the Responses That Maintain the Image

In the sixth step, the client and therapist(s) are trying to find out what the client does when he or she experiences the image, which ultimately maintains it. What the client does in response to the image should make sense, now that the power of the image has been clarified. The response may be an internal action, an observable act, or both. Responses to an image tend to fall into loose categories corresponding to the power attributed to the image, as shown in Table 7.1.

For example, clients who think that an image is real or happening now will act accordingly (e.g., run away from a frightening image—or, more worryingly, start to make a suicide plan for a hopeless future image). For more pleasurable images, clients may stay absorbed in them when they should be doing other things. Whatever the precise response, the clients will be acting as if the content of the image is real, and will not be dismissing it as simply a mental event.

If clients think that an image is prophetic or a warning, they may replay it many times, to try to work out what it is trying to tell them. Alternatively, the client may engage in some "superstitious" act to prevent the image from coming true (e.g., a cognitive ritual), or may even start to prepare for what the image predicts (e.g., a death). Again, the client will respond as if the image is true, rather than just an image inside their heads.

If clients think that holding an image in mind might overwhelm them or make them go mad/collapse, then they may respond by pushing the image away or trying to distract themselves from it. This distraction can range from the mundane (e.g., putting on the television or listening to loud music) to more drastic attempts at avoidance (e.g., substance abuse or deliberate self-harm). Clients will use similar strategies if they think that dwelling on the image might take them back to the past. Alternatively, they may try to anchor themselves in the present, by paying attention to objects in their immediate surroundings or by reciting an anchoring phrase or sentence (e.g., "I am OK; it is 2018; I am in London").

If clients think that an image might affect others, then, logically, they will either attempt to dispel it (using distraction) or undertake superstitious acts to prevent it from coming true (as above).

TABLE 7.1. Likely Client Responses to Mental Images

Power attributed to image in step 5	Likely response to image
The image is real/happening now.	The client behaves as if the image were happening (e.g., runs away from a frightening image, makes a suicide plan for a hopeless image, stays absorbed in a pleasurable image). The client does not dismiss the image, as it is not considered simply to be happening inside his or her head.
The client fears that he or she may go mad, die, collapse, or be overwhelmed if the image stays in mind.	The client attempts to push the image out of his or her mind or to distract him- or herself from the image. Attempts to distract can range from mild attention-switching tasks (e.g., watching TV) to drastic competing tasks (e.g., severe substance misuse or deliberate self-harm).
The image seems like a premonition.	The client may replay the image many times while trying to work out what it is telling him or her and what to do about it. Alternatively, the client may undertake some "superstitious" act to prevent the image from coming true (e.g., retrace steps or perform some cognitive ritual), or a preparatory act to get ready for what is believed will happen (e.g., start to get personal affairs in order for a premonition of death).
The image may affect others.	Generally, the client believes that the image may affect others in a negative way. Thus the client will take steps to dispel the image (as above) or to prevent it from coming true (as above).
Holding the image in mind may take the client back to past/elsewhere.	The client will try to dispel the image (as above) or undertake "grounding" actions to anchor him- or herself in the present (e.g., pay extra attention to current surroundings or recite an anchoring phrase/ sentence). Alternatively, the client may try to change the image to make it less threatening (e.g., by introducing someone or something that anchors them in the present). *Note: Grounding can be seen as an adaptive response to genuine flashbacks in a client with PTSD, so if clients are taking grounding action, it is worth checking that their responses really are maintaining their images/that their images aren't flashbacks.*
Having the image *means* something about the client.	If the client believes that having the image means something bad about him- or herself, the client may withdraw from others or become self-punitive in some way. If the client believes that it means something good about him or her, the client may become excited or grandiose and act accordingly. The client may also try to keep the image in mind or get it to return when it goes.

Finally, if clients think that having an image means something about them, they will respond accordingly. If they think that an image means something negative about them, they may punish themselves or withdraw from others. If they think that it means something positive (e.g., that they are gifted, special, or hyperintelligent), then they may act in an excited or grandiose way.

Clearly, there are a number of possible responses to an image. These responses form the final part of a vicious circle, whereby the image is more likely to persist or to occur again. It is useful to think about *how* a client's response to an image makes the image more likely to persist. A combination of classical/operant conditioning paradigms and some basic cognitive theories of memory can be used to explain this persistence in most cases. These explanations are summarized in Table 7.2.

If clients simply push their images away, then we know that the images will recur because of the classic "thought suppression rebound" effect—the phenomenon whereby trying to stop thinking about something causes a paradoxical increase in its occurrence (see, e.g., Wegner, Schneider, Carter, & White, 1987). However, if clients use self-harm or substance misuse to distract themselves from images, then we hypothesize that the medium-term lowering of mood that follows will make the negative images more accessible, through "mood-dependent memory retrieval" (see, e.g., Lewis & Critchley, 2003).

A similar mechanism is likely to operate when clients act as if an image is real. We hypothesize that this will generate strong image-congruent emotions (e.g., fear in a frightening image or sadness in a hopeless image), which will then make the image more accessible. Mood lowering after self-punishment/withdrawal from others (in the case where clients

TABLE 7.2. How Responses to a Mental Image Reinforce the Image

Response to image	Mechanism of image maintenance
Pushing out	Classic thought suppression rebound effect occurs.
More drastic pushing out (e.g., substance misuse, self-harm)	Medium- to long-term mood lowering retriggers image.
Replaying the image	Image is replayed; emotions intensify.
Acting as if image were real	Such strong image-congruent emotion (e.g., fear) is generated that image is then retriggered.
Superstitious act to avoid premonition	Belief in premonition is not challenged; superstitious act is negatively reinforced; image remains powerful.
Grounding actions to keep from being taken to past/elsewhere	Belief in power of image to take client elsewhere is not challenged; grounding actions are negatively reinforced; image remains powerful.
Belief that image means something bad about self	Withdrawal/self-punishment will lower mood and retrigger image.
Belief that image means something good about self	Excited behavior will induce high mood, retriggering image. Absorption in image will obviously maintain it.

believe that the image means something bad about themselves) will also make the image more likely to be retriggered. Conversely, if clients believe that a positive image means something good about themselves, the resultant good mood will increase the likelihood of the image's persisting. Finally, if clients undertake "grounding" or superstitious acts in response to an image, they will never discover whether or not the image actually *is* as powerful as they fear it is; thus the power of the image remains. Moreover, because the grounding or superstitious act improved their mood, they are more likely to undertake it next time the image occurs (a phenomenon known as "negative reinforcement"; see, e.g., Skinner, 1953).

A therapist might want to introduce this step to a client as follows:

> "So you have told me that you get this image of [details]. When you have it in your mind, you feel [for example] very sad. You are thinking [details], and the image is so clear that you believe [for example] that it must be more than a passing thought, that it is some kind of premonition. Given that, what do you do when the image comes into your mind? Do you try to push it away? Or perhaps replay it in your mind's eye? Do you do something to protect yourself or others from what happens in the image? Or do you do something to help you cope with how the image makes you feel?"

It is also useful to think about not just the client's immediate reaction to the image, but also what further behaviors follow in different contexts and situations. For example, a client who believes that an image may affect others may, in the moment, try to dismiss it. However, he or she may gradually withdraw from others over several weeks or months, in an attempt to protect them.

Step 7: Identify the Triggers and Original Source of the Image

Once the client and therapist(s) understand the image in detail, they should be able to explore together what tends to trigger it. Often a client will know what acts as a trigger. If not, standard antecedent–behavior–consequence (A-B-C) procedures should help. For example, recent occurrences of the image may be examined for patterns of antecedents, and if this doesn't help, diaries can be used. Useful questions might include these:

> "When do you notice the image popping up?"
>
> "Are there any particular situations, places, or thought processes that seem to trigger the image?"
>
> "When and where does the image most frequently come?"

Typical triggers identified by clients have included receiving an invitation to a social event, turning on the computer, or seeing the person about whom they have an image.

In this final step, the client and therapist(s) also look for the original source of the image. Of course, there are many images for which no source can be identified. However, sometimes an image has its roots in a highly emotional or traumatic event. Alternatively, it may just have taken shape over time. Useful questions might include these:

"When was the first time you had this image?"

"Is it linked to something that has happened to you in the past?"

"Is there something in particular it reminds you of?"

What to Do Once the Microformulation Is Complete

Now that the microformulation is complete, the therapist(s) and client need to take some time to look at it together. Are there any bits that don't feel quite right? Do they need to talk some more about any part of it?

Once a target image has been microformulated, the selection of treatment strategy or strategies should be fairly obvious. In the chapters on treatment that follow, we describe the various options and the kinds of microformulations that might lead to the choice of each option. It is worth noting that several different strategies may be useful for one client. Table 7.3 provides a general guide to selecting an imagery treatment strategy after microformulation.

PSYCHOEDUCATION FOR CLIENTS

Before the start of any particular intervention, it is worth introducing the client to the idea of changing or responding differently to the mental image, and to the benefits that this change might bring. Some clients are dubious about the benefits of changing images, particularly with a rescripting that is not real or possible. Equally, while clients may be reacting to images as if they were real, they may not understand why they have been doing this.

Description of Steps

The precise details of a psychoeducation session need to be tailored to the individual client and to the particular techniques the therapist(s) and client may employ together. However, these essential points should be made clear:

1. Imagery has a more powerful impact on emotion than verbal cognition does.
2. Imagery has perceptual equivalence with real experience.
3. Imagery influences learning and behavior.

The discussion should also include how this information from the research world relates to the client's experiences, and how it might be used to help the client in the future.

Scientific Information about Mental Imagery

This discussion needs to be as interactive and interesting as possible. As it is quite lengthy, the therapist(s) should pause regularly and check that the client is following it. In our experience, having psychoeducation information available to look at helps clients to follow what therapists are saying. *We recommend having this section of the manual open on the table, so that everyone can see it as the therapist(s) and client talk.*

A therapist might want to say something like this:

"People often say that imagery has a more powerful effect on your emotions than just thinking in words. Certainly, as we have been discussing your images over the last few weeks, we have found that they can have a profound impact on your mood.

"A group of researchers have found evidence of just how large the impact of imagery on mood can be. We thought it might be quite useful to take you through this research.

TABLE 7.3. Picking an Imagery Treatment Strategy after Microformulation

What microformulation highlights	Treatment strategy to consider
Attention is "hijacked" by distorted imagery that is mistaken for reality.	If the client is overwhelmed by repetitive images to the extent that they impair functioning, the first step may be metacognitive techniques to gain some sense of control.
	Once the client's sense of control is improved, imagery rescripting of the most pertinent image(s) should be considered.
Compelling imagery is capturing attention for sustained periods.	Metacognitive techniques or competing visuospatial tasks.
Imagery does reflect reality, but client needs to spend less time absorbed in it.	Metacognitive techniques.
Unhelpful images are of *actual* past events.	Imagery rescripting techniques.
Unhelpful images are of *imagined* past, current, or future events.	Imagery rescripting techniques.
Unhelpful images are of actual/imagined past, current, or future events, but there are too many such images to rescript each individually.	Positive imagery techniques or metacognitive techniques.
Unhelpful images have their roots in childhood experiences (often traumatic experiences) and are "felt sense" images without a picture that can be rescripted.	Positive imagery techniques.
There is a need to increase the client's ability to self-soothe.	Positive imagery techniques.
Unhelpful images warrant rescripting, but rescripting is not possible at present.	Competing visuospatial tasks.
There is a need for an immediate way to disrupt troubling imagery while further assessment/microformulation takes place.	Competing visuospatial tasks.

"What the researchers wanted to do was to see whether there was any difference between how upset people got if they thought about the same distressing things in words or in images.

"They gave volunteers a series of more than 100 picture–word combinations (each one was a photograph with a word underneath it). Of these combinations, half were benign, such as the picture of a cliff with the word 'view' [shown in Figure 7.2], and half were negative, such as the picture of a cliff with the word 'jump' [shown in Figure 7.3].

"We know from previous research that if you show people lots of distressing materials like the cliff and 'view' combination, by the end of the experiment they could become upset.

"In this experiment, half the participants were asked to 'imagine the combination of the picture and word' (this was called the 'imagery condition'), and the other half were asked to 'make a sentence about the picture and word' (this was called the 'verbal condition'). They were also given a questionnaire, which measured how anxious they were feeling both before and after presentation of all the picture–word combinations. Participants in both groups viewed exactly the same picture–word combinations. So the researchers thought that if there was any difference in how anxious the participants felt at the end of the experiment, it must be the result of whether participants were thinking in images or words.

"The researchers found that when participants thought about the negative picture–word combinations in imagery rather than in words, they were three times more anxious at the end of the experiment. Similarly, when they thought about the benign combinations in imagery rather than in words, they were four times less anxious [as shown in Figure 7.4].

"So this research shows that, just as we suspected, thinking about things in images has a much greater effect on how you feel than thinking about them verbally has. But why? Recent research from neuroscience helps us to explain.

"Brain scientists have used neuroimaging to investigate what is happening when someone imagines something, rather than seeing, hearing, or doing it 'for real.' Participants are put in a brain scanner machine and are either instructed to imagine something

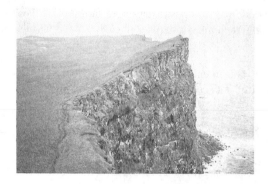

view

FIGURE 7.2. An example of a positive picture–word combination.

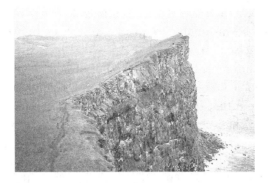

jump

FIGURE 7.3. An example of a negative picture–word combination.

(for example, an angry facial expression) or are presented with the actual thing (for example, a photograph of an angry face). They have done this with imagining/seeing simple pictures, imagining/seeing more complex scenes, imagining/hearing music, and imagining rotating/actually rotating an object. When they compare the brain scans, they find that there is little difference; that is, the scan of someone imagining a tune is almost the same as the scan of someone actually hearing the tune. It is as if the brain can't quite tell the difference between your doing something and your imagining doing something.

"In fact, for studies exploring 'looking at' versus 'imagining' visual materials, the researchers found that in most studies, area 17 of the primary visual cortex in the brain was being activated when visual information was solely being imagined. Area 17 is thought to be the first area of the brain that visual information from outside 'hits' when we look at something in the real world. It seems the brain is responding to an imagined

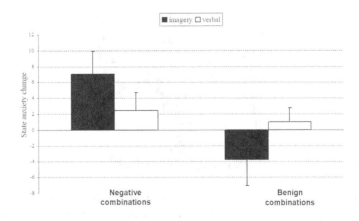

FIGURE 7.4. Changes in state anxiety (on the State–Trait Anxiety Inventory) over negative and benign picture–word combinations for the imagery and verbal conditions. Data from Holmes, Mathews, Mackintosh, and Dalgleish (2008).

picture as if the information is coming from outside the person's head. So, no wonder the brain sometimes seems unable to tell the difference between imagining and actually seeing something [see Figure 7.5]!

"Finally, in another recent study, researchers asked people to imagine increasingly bright lights. The people knew they were imagining; that was all they were being asked to do. The study found that the brighter the lights people were imagining, the more their pupils dilated. Their pupils were behaving as if they were actually seeing the lights for real, even though the people knew that they were only imagining.

"So what does all of this mean for you? It means that when you have a frightening mental image (for instance, of crashing your car), it is likely to make you feel more frightened than if you were thinking about the same thing but in words (for instance, 'What if I crash my car?'). This is probably because your brain is reacting as if you were seeing the frightening thing for real.

"However, not only does the brain respond to the frightening image as if it is real, but it also makes your body react as if the frightening thing were in the room with you. Your heart will race; you might get ready to run away; or you might even freeze and be unable to move at all. This has been demonstrated by researchers in laboratories, but it is also something most of us experience when we have a sexual fantasy. When we fantasize about something sexual, it has a profound effect on our bodies and our minds, even when we know full well that we are just imagining it.

"Furthermore, research has confirmed that not only does mental imagery affect people's bodies, it also has an impact on their behavior. A team of researchers got a group of people with low mood to bring to mind a series of positive images. After doing this, not only had their moods improved, but they performed better when they played a simple game (a children's fishing game). Similarly, we know people who take

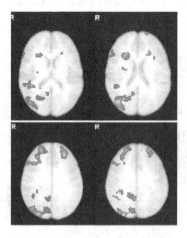

FIGURE 7.5. Pattern of activation of a functional magnetic resonance imaging (fMRI) scan of the brain during a mental imagery task (imagining complex visual scenes). Similar areas are involved in processing external visual complex scenes, exemplifying the major overlaps in brain function during mental imagery and perception. Unpublished fMRI data courtesy of Martina Di Simplicio.

illegal drugs are more likely to do so again after they have experienced positive mental images, anticipating taking the drugs.

"To summarize, what all of this means is that if you are, for example, imagining something frightening, you are likely to feel more frightened than if you were thinking about the same thing but in words. This is because your brain is reacting to the frightening image as if it were real, *and* your body will also react as if you were genuinely in the presence of the frightening thing. This effect is the same for negative and positive or exciting images.

"This research helps to explain why you react as strongly as you do to the mental images we have discussed in recent weeks. However, it also opens up a whole new avenue of things we could do to help you and others like you. For example, if you can convince yourself that something is 'only' an image, and we can find a way to override the brain reacting to it as if it were real, you can see how that might help. Equally, you can deliberately use positive images to induce powerful positive moods. For instance, if you can vividly imagine lying in a gorgeous meadow, on a beautiful day, feeling happy, then your brain may react as if you are actually there and make you feel happy. Finally, if you have upsetting images of things going wrong in the past or future, you can learn to change them, to make the ending better. It doesn't matter if something you imagine is real or possible; as long as you imagine it vividly, your brain can react to the image as if it is real/actually happening, and your mood will change accordingly.

"Sports psychologists have been using this research for many years to improve the performance of athletes. Footballers [or, for U.S. clients, soccer players] rehearse in imagination taking the perfect penalty kick hundreds of times. Each time they rehearse it, their brain is reacting to it as if they have just scored the goal. So, when they come to take the penalty kick, they have the confidence of having essentially scored hundreds of perfect goals. Similarly, divers rehearse their dives in imagination; cricketers [or, for U.S. clients, baseball players] rehearse their swings; and sprinters imagine their record-breaking finishes. Musicians also report practicing their pieces in imagination on their way to a performance, and so on. So, while the power of mental images often ends up being a negative thing, with a bit of thought, we can turn it into a powerful tool for change."

Relating the Research Findings to the Client's Experiences

There is a lot of information to cover here, but we have found that all clients benefit from understanding the science behind the imagery techniques used in this treatment. The psychoeducation also helps to explain why the clients' mental images have been having such a profound impact upon them.

Having checked a client's understanding of the information, the therapist(s) should invite the client to think about how it helps him or her to explain their reaction to the mental images and the impact they have been having upon the client's daily life. The discussion can then move on to consider how the client could harness the power of mental imagery to make things easier in the future.

CLIENT REFLECTIONS ON MICROFORMULATION AND PSYCHOEDUCATION

The following are quotes from MAPP clients who were asked for feedback at the end of treatment. They reflect the usefulness of the insights the clients gained during the microformulation and psychoeducation processes.

"As the sessions unfolded, it became clear that I was a really 'imagey' thinker—something that I was totally oblivious to before MAPP. Honestly, the whole experience was a real eye-opener. I guess that no one thinks about how they think; they just do it because that's what they've always done, and there's never been any reason to engage with it before."

"I always knew I had a powerful visual memory, but I just sort of assumed everyone else was like me. I can recall with almost photographic accuracy many parts of my childhood and school years, and find it fun to indulge in the happier memories."

CONCLUDING COMMENTS

This chapter has covered probably the most important component of the MAPP therapy protocol—the part where the client and therapist(s) start to understand how and why a problematic image is having such an impact on the client's mood. This is done through the process of microformulating the image and then sharing some psychoeducation about the "science" behind the impact of images. In the chapters that follow, we explain how to undertake each of the therapeutic techniques for working with images.

For further reading on the basic science of mental imagery, see Pearson and colleagues (2015), Holmes and Mathews (2005), or Holmes, Mathews, and colleagues (2008).

CHAPTER 8

Metacognitive Techniques to Reduce the Power of the Image

"Metacognitive techniques" are a group of strategies aimed at reducing the emotional power of an image by changing how a client relates to the image. They reinforce that the image is just an image, that the client does not need to pay attention to the image, and that the client should direct his or her attention beyond or outside of the image. In most cases, there is little or no engagement with the content of the image. These techniques are rarely used as the sole treatment, but they can be particularly useful in the following situations:

- When attention is "hijacked" or "captured" by distorted imagery that is mistaken for external reality (e.g., in social anxiety, where distorted images of how clients think they look to other people interfere with their ability to perform socially).
- When compelling imagery captures attention for a sustained period (e.g., "flashforwards" to suicide being played over and over in a client's mind, or images of future successes and possessions). Absorption in such imagery can have a powerful impact on mood, but also can distract clients and even prevent them from undertaking normal daily activities
- When an image does reflect reality (e.g., the person *is* isolated, or a relative *has* died), but the client needs to spend less time absorbed in the image.

In situations like these, clients and therapists develop metacognitive techniques that will help the clients to disengage from the absorbing mental imagery and direct their attention elsewhere.

It is worth noting that metacognitive elements can also be integrated into other treatment techniques, to great effect—for example, as elements of rescripting an image (see Chapter 9).

DESCRIPTION OF STEPS

Effective use of metacognitive techniques can be achieved by following these four steps:

1. Identify the types of situations in which images hijack/capture attention.
2. Microformulate how the attention capture might maintain current difficulties.
3. Check out the microformulation in session.
4. Develop strategies for disengaging from the image and shifting attentional focus in novel situations.

Step 1: Identify the Types of Situations in Which Images Hijack/Capture Attention

A client first carries out monitoring of the treatment target (e.g., social anxiety) between sessions, in order to see whether his or her attention is being captured by mental images and whether this capture may be a factor maintaining the difficulties. For example, the client may record instances of feeling anxious in social situations and notice what images or other thoughts are experienced at these times. These thoughts and images can then be explored in more detail in the session. In the case example provided later in this chapter, the client (Eric) noticed that when he felt anxious in social situations, he had a strong mental image in which he saw other people as far away from him—as if they were being seen through a telescope.

Step 2: Microformulate How the Attention Capture Might Maintain Current Difficulties

In the session, the client and therapist(s) can develop an idiosyncratic microformulation, suggesting how attention capture might play a role in the maintenance of the problem. For Eric, his microformulation suggested that he acted as if the "telescopic" image were true and withdrew from social interaction. This withdrawal meant that he did not find out whether or not he would be able to interact with the others, and thus his anxiety was maintained.

Step 3: Check Out the Microformulation in Session

In the session, the therapist(s) and client can then test the microformulation to see if it is correct. They can carry out experiments to explore the effect on the target problem of attending to internal imagery. For example, if the imagery capturing the client's attention is a distorted representation of reality that then provokes anxiety, the therapist(s) and client can see what happens to the client's anxiety when he or she shifts focus from the mental image to the therapy room. Checking out the microformulation in this way will enhance the credibility of any potential intervention and will start to engender a curious and experimental attitude toward finding ways of dealing with troubling images.

Metacognitive techniques fall into two main categories:

1. *Switching techniques*, in which the client switches the focus of attention from internal images to the outside world. These are very like the grounding techniques used to manage dissociation in PTSD. They work best when the new focus of attention in the outside world is quite absorbing or interesting in its own right.
2. *Image property techniques*, in which the client changes the image in a way that reinforces its unreality.

When introducing these techniques in session, a therapist might want to say something like this:

"As we have already discussed, when you have a vivid mental image, it affects how you feel. We know that for you, your images are so absorbing that you automatically pay attention to them. However, we also know that if you can learn how to disengage from an image that is having a big impact on your mood, it may change your mood. There are various techniques that others have found helpful, and the best way to find out which will work well for you is to try lots of different ones and see how it goes. So we will aim to find a technique or techniques to use when you notice that your attention has been 'captured' by a mental image. It may take us a few weeks of experimentation to find the most effective strategies for different situations."

Examples of each category, and of how to introduce them in session, are provided below.

Switching Techniques

"Can you bring to mind the troubling image? Describe what you can see, hear, smell, and so on. Is that clear in your mind now? Notice how it makes you feel. What emotion are you feeling, or feeling most strongly if there is more than one?

[Client responds.]

"How strong is that [emotion], on a scale where 100% is the strongest it can be and 0% is no emotion?

[Client responds.]

"Let's try shifting your focus. Could you describe for me the objects on the shelf behind my desk? [Other visual options might be to count books on a shelf or look out of the window and notice the colors of cars going by, who is wearing black, who is wearing a hat, or the like.] Try to do this for at least a minute.

[Client responds.]

"Now can you bring your focus back to yourself? [Pause.] How do you feel now? What has happened to the [emotion]? How strong is it now on the scale from 0 to 100%?"

The therapist(s) and client can also try switching to attend to auditory stimuli in the outside world. A therapist might say something like this:

"Can you bring to mind the troubling image? Describe what you can see, hear, smell, and so on. Is that clear in your mind now? Notice how it makes you feel. What emotion are you feeling, or feeling most strongly if there is more than one?

[Client responds.]

"How strong is that [emotion], on a scale where 100% is the strongest it can be and 0% is no emotion?

[Client responds.]

"Let's try shifting your focus. Listen for a few seconds and tell me what you hear. Focus on the sounds around us, even things you hear outside, and tell me what you hear.

[Client responds.]

[Therapist asks further questions, such as how many different engine sounds client can hear, or whether client can describe the sensory qualities of others' speech.]

[Client responds.]

"Now can you bring your focus back to yourself? [Pause.] How do you feel now? What has happened to the [emotion]? How strong is it now on the scale from 0 to 100%?"

This exercise can then be repeated with smell and touch, to see which sensory modality is the most effective for the client. For smell, the therapist(s) can provide a range of different-smelling oils/perfumes (in bottles or on pieces of tissue paper) for the client to smell and describe. Similarly, for touch, the therapist(s) can encourage the client to feel and describe materials with different textures, such as the fabric on the client's chair, a rough stone or shell, a "squeezy stress" ball, a lump of clay, or a strip of Velcro. However, if the client has been persuaded of the benefits of switching attention and is keen on using (for instance) visual switching, then there is no need to do more.

Image Property Techniques

"Can you bring to mind the troubling image? Describe what you can see, hear, smell, and so on. Is that clear in your mind now? Notice how it makes you feel. What emotion are you feeling, or feeling most strongly if there is more than one?

[Client responds.]

"How strong is that [emotion] out of 100%, on a scale where 100% is the strongest it can be and 0% is no emotion?

[Client responds.]

"Now I want you to imagine popping the image like a balloon. Can you do that? [Pause.] Tell me what is happening.

[Client responds.]

"How do you feel now? What has happened to the [emotion]? How strong is it now on the scale from 0 to 100%?

[Client responds.]

"Let's try some other techniques until we find that one that works the best for you.

"Can you bring to mind the troubling image? Describe what you can see, hear, smell, and so on. Is that clear in your mind now? Notice how it makes you feel. What emotion are you feeling, or feeling most strongly if there is more than one?

[Client responds.]

"How strong is that [emotion] out of 100%, on a scale where 100% is the strongest it can be and 0% is no emotion?

[Client responds.]

"Now I want you to imagine smashing the image like glass. Can you do that? [Pause.] Tell me what is happening.

[Client responds.]

"How do you feel now? What has happened to the [emotion]? How strong is it now on the scale from 0 to 100%?"

[Client responds.]

The therapist(s) can go through more options to find the most effective one(s). Other options that we found useful in the MAPP case series included these:

- Imagining shrinking the image or blowing it up.
- Imagining the image on a TV screen and turning it off, turning down the volume, or pressing the mute button.
- Imagining the image on a smartphone screen and swiping it to the side.
- Changing the color of the image.
- Imagining making the image look funny (e.g., putting a red nose on someone, or funny clothes).
- Imagining putting the image in a bottle and throwing it out to sea.
- Imagining putting the image on a page in a book and then turning the page over.

Step 4: Develop Strategies for Disengaging from the Image and Shifting Attentional Focus in Novel Situations

In-session experimentation will provide some ideas for how a client might be able to shift attention from unhelpful internal imagery. However, which strategies work best will vary considerably from person to person and from situation to situation. Thus clients need to carry out some experimentation between sessions, to find what methods work best for them in different circumstances in the "real world." Therapists should encourage clients to practice between sessions, noticing the impact of each strategy they try on their ability to shift focus and on their mood. Having clients keep records of this experimentation over a week or two should enable them and their therapists to work together on identifying the most effective strategies.

It would also be sensible to encourage clients to continue informally monitoring the use of the strategies and their real-world effectiveness, and to use what they learn from this monitoring to refine them over the course of therapy and beyond.

CASE EXAMPLE: ERIC

Eric reported social anxiety in relation to joining in conversations with groups of people at social occasions (e.g., at parties, in conversations with other parents at the school gate, and during his lunch break at work). Through his keeping a diary of spontaneous images that arose in these situations, he and his therapists identified that he experienced a distorted visual image of the scene, such that the group of people looked far away—"as if I were looking through a telescope the wrong way around," or "as if they were hazy mirages in a desert." Eric then noticed that this image made him feel anxious and hopeless, as it increased his sense of other people being distant and unreachable and of him being separate from them. (See Eric's completion of a modified Microformulation Template in Figure 8.1.) Because he responded to the image as if it were real, he held back from joining in the groups. Sadly, this then reinforced his view that he was a social failure, and thus heightened his anxiety in social situations.

Experimenting with focusing on this distorted image in session provided support for its role in increasing Eric's anxiety. Eric and his therapists were then able to practice switching from this distorted image to the external scene (gazing around the therapy room, counting the books on the shelf), which resulted in reduced anxiety. Through repeated monitoring and experimentation between sessions, Eric expanded this basic strategy across a range of other anxiety-provoking situations. He would notice that he was having the image, and then refocus on the external scene. For example, when he was outside, Eric would focus on what people were wearing on their heads; when he was inside, he would notice all the things of a particular color in the room.

Hints and Tips for Using Metacognitive Techniques

For three reasons, it is important that a client be engaged in the process of discovering and refining strategies to redirect attention when it has been hijacked by mental imagery. First, the most helpful strategies may be highly idiosyncratic and need to be discovered through experimentation, rather than imposed from a therapist's standard "toolkit." Second, a client who is truly engaged in the process of discovery is much more likely to be interested in the process and motivated to discover, test, and refine the most useful strategies. A self-discovered and self-developed strategy may be much more memorable than one that has been taught by a therapist. Third, discussing the data recorded by the client between sessions (and deciding how to refine techniques on the basis of it) is a useful way to demonstrate to the client the importance of this kind of careful monitoring. It also provides a model for the client him- or herself to develop the strategy beyond the sessions.

If a client's level of engagement seems low, then it is worth stopping and addressing the issue. In the MAPP case series, we found the following helpful when engagement seemed poor:

- First, we would bring up the concern and ask our clients if they agreed.
- Together, we would think about possible next steps: doing chair work, or reviewing the psychoeducation, or revising the microformulation (if it still did not feel right to a client).
- If all else failed, we would suggest trying one of the metacognitive techniques anyway, "just in case" they might help. Because the techniques generally did help reduce the emotion in a troubling image, this demonstration would then increase engagement.

Original source

Possibly an upsetting incident that occurred
when Eric was on a school trip at age 16.

Trigger(s)

Seeing (for example) colleagues together,
having an informal chat.

Image description

Seeing colleagues as small, far away,
at the end of a telescope, unreachable;
sense of self as separated from others
(far away, like a mirage in the desert).

**Maintaining factors
for persistence of image**

Act on what is seen in the
image: distance. Walk away,
stand apart.

**Emotion(s)
in image**

Anxiety

Low mood

**Appraisal(s)
in image**

"Should I join them?
I won't belong."

"I'm a social failure."

**Power of the image:
Why is it not dismissed?**

Image feels very real and is not
appraised as an image at the time.

Notice having an image. Pause and
make a conscious choice, rather than
automatically going along with the
image and its meaning. Use switching
techniques, such as noticing colors or
headgear.

Greater social interaction; reduction
in negative image intrusions.

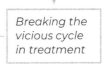

Breaking the
vicious cycle
in treatment

FIGURE 8.1. Eric's filled-in Microformulation Template (Appendix 4, somewhat modified/stream-lined for illustrative purposes), describing the etiology and maintenance of his target disruptive imagery. A potential "escape route" or way to break the cycle of intrusive imagery is indicated via use of a meta-cognitive technique.

CLIENT REFLECTION ON METACOGNITIVE TECHNIQUES

The following is a quote from a MAPP client who was asked for feedback at the end of treatment. It reflects the usefulness of the metacognitive technique that this client, who was often an unwilling witness to arguments between other people, learned to use.

> "A great idea I got from MAPP was that I could treat everything that was going on in my head like a scene from a film I was watching. So I learned to become more like a spectator of the scene, rather than being one of the key actors. I pulled the 'camera' away from the first-person perspective, and moved it to a different place in the room. This simple switch, surprisingly, immediately separated me from the strong emotions in that room. I could see myself sitting there, watching . . . and could listen to the fight going on in the room without becoming anxious and upset. Another time, I tried to remove the camera completely: I took the camera, left the room, and closed the door behind me, leaving the fight and the emotions in there. I let that imaginary door close behind me, and then the voices became muffled . . . what a relief! Once I got it, I was able to advance this technique in any way that I figured out could help put further distance between me and any upsetting situations I was embroiled in! For example, I was taught to place the entire event onto a screen, as if I were watching it at a cinema; I would even put myself in the cinema, as a viewer. Then I figured out I could simply watch myself get up and walk out of the cinema . . . and just let go. Eventually I would picture myself walking away down the road on a warm, sunny day, leaving the stress and angst of the situation playing away on that distant cinema screen."

CONCLUDING COMMENTS

In this chapter, we have covered how to introduce and work with metacognitive techniques. While these techniques are quite simple to learn and implement, they nevertheless form an important part of most imagery-based interventions. They teach clients the crucial lesson that a very troubling image is just a mental event, and they do not necessarily have to attend to it and experience the emotions within it.

In the next chapter, we describe how to use the next most frequently used imagery technique: imagery rescripting.

CHAPTER 9

Imagery Rescripting Techniques

Imagery rescripting can be used with images of actual events from the past or with fictional past, current, or future events. The overall aim of rescripting is simple: to change how the image makes the client *feel* and/or how the client *reacts to it*. This is a very important point to remember; what is happening within a mental image is interesting, but how it makes our clients *feel or act* is where we need to direct our attention as therapists. Changing how an image makes someone feel or act will, in turn, alter the mood-destabilizing effect of the image.

RATIONALE FOR IMAGERY RESCRIPTING

The rationale for imagery rescripting techniques is probably best explained while the therapist(s) and client are looking at the client's microformulation. A therapist might want to say something like this:

> "So we can see that when this image comes to mind, it is associated with a whole host of emotions and meanings that have a big impact on you and lead you to do X. In order to change this impact, we need to counter the 'toxicity' of the meaning with an 'antidote.' We are carefully going to work through what we need for this antidote image to make it work well. Then we will practice replacing the old toxic image with the new antidote image, checking that the new image makes you feel better and that you don't need to do X. Eventually, you should be able to replace the old image with the new one whenever it comes to mind."

DESCRIPTION OF STEPS

Imagery rescripting can be achieved through following these five steps:

1. Describe the emotions and appraisals contained in the original image (its meaning).
2. Find the opposite meaning (the antidote).
3. Create an image that represents the antidote.
4. Go back to the original image and hold it in mind.
5. Insert the antidote image when affect is "hot" (intense).

These steps are shown in diagrammatic form in Figure 9.1.

Throughout this chapter, we use the example of a client named Sameena, who had a "flashforward" of herself performing badly in a work meeting. She described the image as follows:

> "I am sitting in the meeting room, the one we always use. It is a large room with big windows down the left-hand side. There is a U-shaped table, and there are half a dozen of us sitting there, with my line manager, Martha, behind a smaller table at the front. Sunlight is streaming in through the window—it feels hot and stuffy. . . . I am sitting right at the bottom of the U, opposite Martha. I can see the image through my own eyes. I can hear people coughing nervously and someone tapping their pencil against the table on my right . . . it's so loud . . . it is echoing. Everyone is looking at me. I am holding my notes in my right hand. Martha is waiting for me to start describing my report, but I can't, I can't read it out. . . . I feel hotter and hotter. I can feel that my face is shiny. I can't breathe. Everyone is looking at me with pity . . . they can see I am blanking."

What follows is a step-by-step guide for how to rescript an image. Clinicians more experienced in working with imagery may be able to move from the meaning of the troublesome image to developing an antidote image quickly. It should not feel arduous, so there is no need to go through all of these stages (i.e., working with a client to complete all of the charts we describe below) if a therapist and client feel able to move more rapidly. The details below are for readers who are less familiar with using imagery.

Step 1: Describe the Emotions and Appraisals Contained in the Original Image (Its Meaning)

In the first step, the therapist(s) and client use the microformulation as a starting point to focus discussion. They will need to refer back to the Chart for Recording Emotions and Appraisals within a Troublesome Image, which they have completed together during microformulation (see Appendix 5 for a blank version). Sameena's completed chart is shown in Figure 9.2.

When we talk about the "meaning" of an image, we are often referring simply to the appraisals the person is making, such as Sameena's appraisal "I am never going to make it in this field." However, sometimes the meaning can also incorporate some elements of the power of the image and the emotions the client experiences when he or she gets the image, such as the following: "I am definitely going to mess this up. I feel so anxious I can't think. This image is so clear, it will come true. It shows the future I am creating. I will not make it in this field."

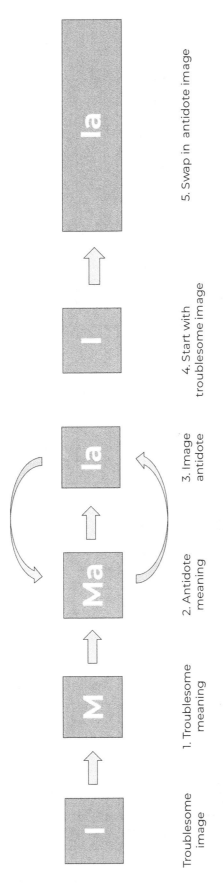

FIGURE 9.1. Flow diagram representing the five steps in rescripting a troublesome mental image.

97

For the target image, fill in the emotion(s) that you feel while you hold it in mind. Then establish what you are thinking/what is running through your mind that is making you feel that emotion. Ensure that you establish this information for *all* of the emotions that you feel when you hold the image in mind.

Image	Emotions: "How do you feel?"	Appraisals: "When you feel X, what is running through your mind? What are you thinking that is making you feel X?"
Image of me sitting in a meeting room, struggling to read my report.	Anxiety	*I am messing this up.*
	Despair	*I am never going to make it in this field.*

FIGURE 9.2. Sameena's filled-in Chart for Recording Emotions and Appraisals within a Troublesome Image (Appendix 5).

The meaning the person ascribes to the image will then, in turn, affect the emotions that he or she feels while experiencing the image, and hence its power. So there is a fluid and mutually excitatory interaction among all of these elements, as shown in Figure 9.3. *This combination of the appraisals, emotions, and power, together making the meaning of an image, explains the impact of the image on the client and why the client reacts to it as he or she does.*

Given that the aim is to change the impact of an image through rescripting, the therapist(s) and client need to make sure that they clearly understand the meaning of each image. We find that it helps to use a worksheet with an additional column to begin the process of rescripting. This is the Chart for Recording the Meaning of a Troublesome Image (see Appendix 6 for a blank version). Sameena's completed chart is shown in Figure 9.4.

The inclusion of ratings (which also distinguishes Appendix 6 from Appendix 5) will help the therapist(s) and client to see how strongly the client believes a given meaning. It is also useful for monitoring change over time. The ratings should refer to the intensity of the emotions and the believability of the meanings when the image is *in the person's mind*—not later, on reflection.

In Sameena's case, one of the meanings ascribed to the image ("This image is so clear, it will come true. It shows the future I am creating. I will not make it in this field") has elements of how the image made her feel (despair), her appraisal ("I'm never going to make it in this field"), *and* the power she ascribed to the image (the fact that the image was so clear that it must be prophetic). Because she had this pessimistic image *and* she believed it to be a prophecy, we can understand why she reacted in that way that she did to it (she despaired and avoided meetings and briefings as much as possible).

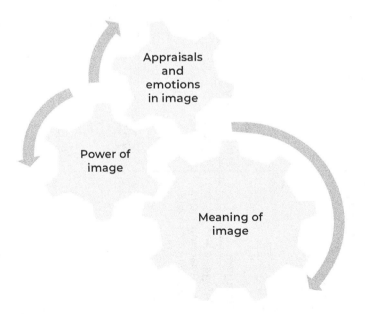

FIGURE 9.3. Diagram showing the mutually excitatory relationship among the meaning, the power, and the appraisals/emotions in a mental image.

For the target image, transfer information (gained during the microformulation stage) into this chart about the emotions and appraisals in the image. Then rate the intensity of the emotions (0–100%). Finally, think about the meaning of the image—the combination of how it makes you feel, what you are thinking, and the power of the image. Together, these things form the meaning of the image and will explain why you react to it in the way that you do. Rate how much you believe this meaning (0–100%) while the image is in your mind, not how much you believe it later.

Image	Emotions: "How do you feel?"	Appraisals: "When you feel X, what is running through your mind? What are you thinking that is making you feel X?" Rate intensity of emotions: 0% (no emotion)–100% (most intense emotions ever experienced).	Meanings: "What is it that you believe or know or feel that explains the way you react to the image?" Rate how much you believe each meaning: 0% (do not believe at all)–100% (completely believe).
Image of me sitting in a meeting room, struggling to read my report.	Anxiety	I am messing this up. (100%)	I am definitely going to mess this up. I feel so anxious I can't think. (100%)
	Despair	I am never going to make it in this field. (90%)	This image is so clear, it will come true. It shows the future I am creating. I will not make it in this field. (90%)

FIGURE 9.4. Sameena's filled-in Chart for Recording the Meaning of a Troublesome Image (Appendix 6).

To help a client think about the "Meanings" column of Appendix 6, it might be useful to say something like the following:

> "We know that when you have this image, it makes you feel *X*, and *Y* is running through your mind. Because of the power of the image, you are also thinking/feeling *Z*. So if we put this all together, we would have the meaning of the image for you and the explanation of why you react in the way that you do. How could we summarize this meaning? What is it that you believe or know or feel that explains the way you react to the image?"

Occasionally, the client will simply restate the appraisals in the image in answer to questions about meaning (e.g., "It means that I will never make it in this field"). We suggest discussing it further, as demonstrated by the following therapeutic dialogue with Sameena.

THERAPIST: When you have the image, you feel sad and despairing. You are thinking, "I am messing this up, and I am never going to make it in this field." So no wonder you are feeling sad and despairing. However, we know that you are really, really sure about the prediction of your failure (90–100%). You are not thinking, "This is just an image—it doesn't mean anything. I am just worrying." You are so sure that you have stopped going to meetings, even though you are getting into trouble, as attending these meetings is a core requirement of your job role. Why is that? Why are you so sure, when you have the image in mind, that it is true?

SAMEENA: Hmm . . . well, I don't question it. Why don't I? . . . hmm . . . I don't know, good question! I guess it is because it is so clear. I can hear the tapping and coughing, I feel hot . . . it doesn't feel like a simple passing thought. . . . It *is* the future, it must be . . . it is so vivid, clear, and strong.

THERAPIST: That makes sense. It feels stronger than normal thoughts . . . so it must be true . . . this image of failure will happen. So that's the meaning the image has for you—not just what you see and hear and feel and think within the image, but that fact that it is definitely going to happen. Not going to meetings, even though it is getting you into trouble, makes perfect sense then, doesn't it? There's no point in going, because you are definitely going to fail anyway.

SAMEENA: Yes, that must be it, but I had never really realized why. I was just reacting to the image, to the future I could see.

THERAPIST: Yes . . . that's the thing about these powerful mental images; they are quick, and often you don't even realize that you have had them . . . they are automatic. But your brain has reacted to them as if they are real, and you act accordingly.

Step 2: Find the Opposite Meaning (the Antidote)

In the second step, the therapist(s) and client jointly construct an antidote or countermeaning to the original meaning (or to each original meaning, if there is more than one). This is a little like thought challenging in standard CBT, but it does not rely as heavily upon concrete external evidence.

A therapist might want to introduce this step to the client as follows:

"When your image comes to mind, as we have seen, it is associated with a whole host of emotions and meanings that have a big impact on you. In order to change this impact, we need to counter the 'toxicity' of the meaning with an 'antidote,' the same way we would use an antidote to counteract a real poison if you had accidentally taken one."

So, for each of the meanings identified, the client should be asked to come up with an antidote. Here are some useful questions that a therapist can ask to help the client with this process:

"What would you have to know/see to change the meaning—not to feel X any more?"

"When you have this image in your mind, and it feels like X, what would be the exact opposite of this meaning?"

"When you have this image in your mind, and it feels like X, what would be a more helpful meaning so you wouldn't feel X any more?"

"What would you have to know/see to feel the opposite of this meaning?"

"What would be helpful to know/feel so that you didn't have to react in the way that you do at the moment?"

For self-critical images, the following questions might be particularly helpful:

"If a compassionate friend were with you, what do you imagine this friend might say as an antidote to this meaning?"

"What would you say to a child or someone you cared about if this person were thinking this about him- or herself?"

Sometimes several countermeanings may be needed for each separate problematic meaning identified. A therapist can prompt a client by asking, "Is there anything else that you think you would need to let yourself know [in the countermeaning] for you to feel OK?"

Note that an antidote may need to encompass all aspects of a problematic meaning—that is, emotions, appraisals, and the perceived power of the image. For Sameena, the antidote needed to (1) counter her feelings of sadness and anxiety (which were caused by her unhelpful appraisals about being a failure and never succeeding in her field); and (2) address her appraisal that this failure was *definitely* going to happen, because her image of it was so vivid.

Helping a client complete the Chart for Constructing an Antidote for a Troublesome Image can be beneficial. (See Appendix 7 for a blank version of this chart.) Sameena's completed chart is shown in Figure 9.5. In completing this chart, the therapist(s) and client focus on the emotions and the toxic meanings, looking for antidote emotions and meanings.

Unlike standard CBT thought challenging, this process is not overly concerned with challenging unhelpful appraisals. This is because a therapist simply wants to change how an image makes a client *feel* and *act*. Sometimes, to achieve this, the therapist will challenge

For the target image, transfer information into this chart about the emotions and meanings in the image. Then think about what emotions would be the opposites/the "antidotes" to the "toxic" emotions. Next, think about what meanings would generate those antidote emotions. Remember, you may need to address all aspects of a toxic meaning with an antidote: toxic emotions, toxic appraisals, and the perceived power of the image. Rate how much you believe the antidote meanings (0–100%). Finally, generate an antidote image to try out—one that encapsulates the antidote meanings and generates the antidote emotions.

Image	Emotions: How do you feel?	Meanings: What is it that you believe or know or feel that explains the way you react to the image? Rate how much you believe each meaning: 0% (do not believe at all)–100% (completely believe).	Antidote Emotions: What would be the antidote to that feeling?	Antidote Meanings: What would you have to know to experience this antidote feeling? (Note: This needs to counter all of the meaning, including the power of the image.) Rate how much you believe each antidote meaning: 0% (do not believe at all)–100% (completely believe).	Antidote Image: What image springs to mind/can we construct that incorporates the antidote meaning and will make you feel the antidote emotions?
Image of me sitting in a meeting room, struggling to read my report.	Anxiety	I am definitely going to mess this up. I feel so anxious I can't think. (100%)	Calm	It is neither big nor clever to always start reporting first. I wait for others to kick off, and listen while looking intelligent and thoughtful and enigmatic. (60%)	I swipe out the old image with my finger, like I'm using a tablet or smartphone. A new image comes in.. I look thoughtful; I am nodding. I feel serene, cool. My heart isn't racing. I don't have to go first at reporting if I don't want to. I look enigmatic, and I feel calm.
	Despair	This image is so clear, it will come true. It shows the future I am creating. I will not make it in this field. (90%)	Hopeful	This is just an image, nothing more. I am making steady progress in this field. (80%)	I swipe backward and forward between this antidote image and the old one, very quickly, several times. See, it's just an image, nothing more. I am making steady progress in this field.

FIGURE 9.5. Sameena's filled-in Chart for Constructing an Antidote for a Troublesome Image (Appendix 7).

appraisals; however, often this is not necessary. Remember, the image itself is the target, rather than the verbal thoughts.

As mentioned previously, clinicians more experienced in using imagery may be able to move from a troublesome image to an antidote image very rapidly. Specifically, they may be able to get to the point of having a description of the image and its associated meaning very quickly (step 1 above), and then be able to help a client to generate an antidote meaning and antidote image simultaneously (steps 2 and 3 combined).

Some people may come up with an antidote meaning very quickly. For others, some Socratic dialogue may be necessary; it may depend upon how strongly they believe the meaning of the image when they do not have it in mind. In Sameena's case, for example, when she had the image in mind, she completely believed it. However, when it was no longer in her mind, Sameena was able to look at her situation more objectively and think about it in a calmer way. She knew that she wasn't doing really badly, relative to the others in her workplace. So she had enough immediate belief in the antidote meaning ("I am making steady progress in this field").

Occasionally, when constructing countermeanings, clients adopt an overly perfectionist stance toward themselves. For example, for the meaning "I'm letting people down," a client may come up with the countermeaning "I will work much harder and then never let people down." In such a case, we suggest guiding the client toward a more balanced, self-compassionate countermeaning, such as "Not responding to a few emails right away does not mean I'm letting people down."

At the end of the session, the therapist(s) should give the client a copy of the antidote meaning or meanings they have constructed together. Usually the meanings will be written in words on a piece of paper or a postcard, but sometimes clients may wish to draw something immediately, or to record their voices in the session. Generally, it is best just to give a client a copy of the antidote meanings, not the affect-laden original meanings. For homework, the client can be asked to read through the countermeanings several times and start to think about the types of positive images, or adaptive changes to the current image, that could capture these new meanings.

Step 3: Create an Image That Represents the Antidote

In the third step, the therapist(s) will help the client to create and to try out the antidote image (or images) in the session a few times—bringing it to mind and then seeing how it makes the client feel. The aim is to ensure that the image encapsulates the antidote meaning and helps the client to feel the antidote emotions.

Ideally, the client will have come to this session with some ideas for the antidote image(s). If so, clearly, it is best to go with the client's images. However, it is worth checking that an image will incorporate all aspects of the antidote meaning. The best way to check this is to get the client to bring the new image to mind, describe it in detail, and then check how it makes the client feel ("Does it elicit all the antidote emotions you were after?") and what it makes the client want to do ("Does it break the vicious circle in the microformulation in the way you want it to?") As the therapist(s) and client do this exercise together, they may find that the image needs to be tweaked.

Occasionally, the client has not been able to come up with an antidote image or images. If this happens, the therapist(s) can try providing some examples of rescripted images others have found helpful. We have had clients with frightening images imagine being able, miraculously, to escape from danger. We have had clients imagine having magic weapons and special powers to do whatever they want to do to feel better. Some clients imagine famous people, spirits, God/gods, and even their therapists making them feel better in their antidote images. Other clients simply change their images to something entirely unrelated that happens to make them feel good. Alternatively, therapists should feel free to suggest things to clients. Clients are generally happy to say so when these suggestions do not feel right. If clients are not sure what they think about a suggestion, they can bring it to mind, elaborate on it, and then see how it makes them feel.

Clients should be reminded as necessary that an antidote image does not have to be real. It simply needs to be more helpful than the troublesome image—to make them feel better than that image does (see the "Hints and Tips . . ." box below for more ideas). Therapists can refer back to earlier discussions about the power of images to make people feel strong emotions, and can add that this works for both "realistic" and "unrealistic" images.

With Sameena, when she brought the antidote image to mind, her therapist checked that it really did make her feel calm, that her heart was not racing, and that she did not think she was not going to fail in her career.

Asking the client to rate the intensity of the antidote emotion should provide accurate information about how well the antidote is working. This exercise should be repeated two or three times in session, to make sure the image is well rehearsed. See the dialogue below for how this was done with Sameena (and refer again to her completed Chart for Constructing an Antidote for a Troublesome Image in Figure 9.5).

THERAPIST: So did you come up with any ideas about what antidote images we could try out today?

SAMEENA: I have got a few ideas. Really, I thought that if I just saw myself as looking thoughtful and serene and intelligent, that might do it.

THERAPIST: Sounds sensible. . . . So this would be how you look to others from an "observer" perspective, as we call it?

SAMEENA: Yes.

THERAPIST: Shall we just try it and see how it makes you feel? Can you close your eyes and bring to mind this new antidote image? Tell me what is happening in this image.

SAMEENA: I can see myself sitting in the room. I am nodding; I look thoughtful.

THERAPIST: What else is happening in the image? What can you hear?

SAMEENA: The same sounds as before—coughing and tapping.

THERAPIST: As you hold that in mind, how does it make you feel? What emotions do you feel?

SAMEENA: Hmm . . . a bit better . . . a bit more calm.

THERAPIST: I wonder how we could make you feel calmer? Maybe it is hard because you are not inside your own body. How about we try the same scene, but this time you are in your own body, nodding and putting a thoughtful expression on your face?

SAMEENA: OK, now I am in my own body. I can see Martha; I can hear the others coughing and tapping. I feel cool and calm. I have that thoughtful expression on my face. I can feel my eyebrows going up into that expression. I know that I look intelligent.

THERAPIST: How do your heart and body feel?

SAMEENA: Calm and cool . . . my heart isn't racing.

THERAPIST: Just focus on that image for a moment. You look intelligent, your body is cool. . . . (*Pause.*) How vivid is the image out of 100%?

SAMEENA: About 60%.

THERAPIST: Keep focusing on it. You look intelligent, your body is cool. . . . (*Pause.*) What emotions do you feel?

SAMEENA: Calm, not anxious.

THERAPIST: Can you rate the calmness out of 100%?

SAMEENA: About 45%.

THERAPIST: Hmm . . . that's actually lower than your first rating. What do you think we need to make you feel less anxious, calmer? What do you need to know or see?

SAMEENA: Hmm . . . maybe something about how that other image is not true, not a prophecy?

THERAPIST: Yes, that sounds important. What would you need to see or do or say to yourself, to know for sure that the pessimistic one was just an image?

SAMEENA: I think I can just say that to myself . . . yes, I am sitting there nodding, looking intelligent and serene, and I am thinking to myself, "That other one was just an image."

THERAPIST: Focus on that for a minute. (*Pause.*) How do you feel now? How calm and not anxious?

SAMEENA: Hmm . . . still only about 50%. When I talk about the other image, it sort of pops into my mind and makes me feel anxious again.

THERAPIST: Ah, so maybe we need to try something that you can do within your antidote image if the old toxic one pops in. People sometimes find it useful to smash the old one like glass, or swipe it away like a smartphone screen, or shrink it. Why not try each one and see which works best? So bring back to mind your new image. There you are, serene and intelligent . . . nodding your head . . . feeling calm and cool. As soon as the toxic image pops in, try one of the techniques I just described to get rid of it.

SAMEENA: OK, there I am feeling calm . . . and in it pops. I have swiped it away . . . it has gone away . . . wow!

THERAPIST: How do you feel?

SAMEENA: Good. That really worked!

THERAPIST: Fantastic! Do you want to try any of the other techniques too (shrink it or smash it), to see which is best?

SAMEENA: No . . . that was brilliant . . . and I don't like the sound of the other ones.

THERAPIST: OK, let's try that one again. Bring to mind the antidote, and then swipe away the old one when it comes. Can you see the antidote? Tell me what's happening.

SAMEENA: There I am, looking calm . . . and in pops the old one . . . I swipe it, it has gone.

THERAPIST: What can you see now?

SAMEENA: Just the antidote.

THERAPIST: How do you feel, and how sure are you that it is worth attending work meetings in the future?

SAMEENA: I feel calm . . . 70% . . . and, yes, I'm fairly sure I should keep on with my career.

THERAPIST: Brilliant! Let's just do it a few times more, to check that it really is working.

Once an antidote image shows promise, the therapist(s) and client may want to use the Chart for Monitoring Progress in Practicing an Antidote Image as they practice it a few times. (See Appendix 8 for a blank version of this chart.) Sameena's completed version of this chart appears in Figure 9.6.

In addition to using ratings of emotion intensity and vividness, a therapist can generally determine that affect shift is occurring by watching a client's posture and noting the tone of voice; these will often change as the client experiences the antidote emotion(s).

In our experience, the "right" antidote image generally begins to produce affect change quite quickly, so only a few practice rounds should be needed in session. If the affect change is not happening, then the therapist(s) and client may need to retrace their steps in generating the antidote image, to try some different things.

When the client has rehearsed the image a few times, and both client and therapist(s) are confident that it is engendering antidote emotions, then they can move on to the next step. If they are not sure, the therapist(s) can ask the client to practice generating the antidote image for homework.

Steps 4 and 5: Go Back to the Original Image and Hold It in Mind; Insert the Antidote Image When Affect is "Hot"

In the last two steps, the aim is to help the client learn to swap the new antidote image for the old, troublesome one. First, the therapist(s) and client do it in session together; then the client can practice it for homework. Eventually, the client needs to be able to swap the antidote for the toxic image in all types of situations in everyday life.

Write a brief description of the antidote image, and then rate (on a scale of 0–100%) the intensity of the antidote emotions generated as you practice the antidote image. Also rate how vivid the image is, on the same scale.

Antidote Image	Antidote Emotions and Vividness Rate intensity of antidote emotions and vividness of image: 0–100%.		
	Practice 1	Practice 2	Practice 3
I swipe out the old image with my finger, like I'm using a tablet or smartphone. A new image comes in. I look thoughtful; I am nodding. I feel serene, cool. My heart isn't racing. I don't have to go first at reporting if I don't want to. I look enigmatic, and I feel calm. I swipe backward and forward between this antidote image and the old one, very quickly, several times. See, it's just an image, nothing more. I am making steady progress in this field.	Calm. Intensity: 70% Hopeful. Intensity: 60% Vividness: 80%	Calm. Intensity: 75% Hopeful. Intensity: 70% Vividness: 90%	Calm. Intensity: 85% Hopeful. Intensity: 70% Vividness: 90%

FIGURE 9.6. Sameena's filled-in Chart for Monitoring Progress in Practicing an Antidote Image (Appendix 8).

This process starts with getting the client to (1) bring to mind the old image; (2) wait until the emotion or emotions in the image are intense (but not too intense—say, 70% of whatever the client considers maximum intensity); and then (3) ask the client to substitute the antidote image(s). This may take some practice. Once an antidote image has been swapped in, a therapist asks the client to describe what he or she can see: Does it engender the antidote emotion? How vivid is it? Is anything else needed in the image—anything else that could help the client to feel the antidote emotion?. If the client is finding it hard to do this swap, a therapist can help by describing the antidote image and encouraging the client to see and hear and feel what the therapist is describing. The dialogue below demonstrates how this was done in session with Sameena.

> THERAPIST: OK, so now that we are happy with the antidote image, we need to practice being able to swap it into your mind when you experience the toxic image in everyday life. The first stage is to do that together. I know we have done it a little when the toxic image "pops" into your antidote—but this time I want us to deliberately bring to mind the toxic image, allow you to feel the emotions in it (say, to about 70% intensity—not the most intense ever), and then swap in the antidote. OK? Can you close your eyes and bring to mind the toxic image, and describe to me what is happening?

> SAMEENA: I am sitting in the room. I can see the windows and Martha and my other colleagues. I can hear coughing and tapping. Everyone is staring at me; they look uncomfortable, pitying. I feel hot. Everyone is looking at me. I am holding my notes in my hand. Martha is waiting for me to start the report, but I can't, I can't read. . . . I can feel that my face is shiny. I can't breathe. Everyone is looking at me with pity . . . they can see I am blanking.

> THERAPIST: How do you feel?

> SAMEENA: Argh . . . terrible . . . hopeless, anxious.

> THERAPIST: How intense out of 100% are those feelings?

> SAMEENA: Bad . . . 70–80%.

> THERAPIST: OK, now swap in the antidote image, and tell me what happens.

> SAMEENA: It's hard, it won't go away . . . it won't budge.

> THERAPIST: It's OK, take your time, we will find a way . . . just describe to me what is happening.

> SAMEENA: I am trying to swipe it, but it won't go.

> THERAPIST: OK, maybe we need to try to tune down the emotion a little in the toxic image. Can you try to turn the image to black and white first, or turn the volume down like with a TV, and then do the swipe? (*Pause.*) Does that help?

> SAMEENA: Yes, that worked better . . . I turned it black and white.

> THERAPIST: OK, let's go on. You have swiped in the antidote image. Tell me what is happening.

SAMEENA: I look thoughtful; I am nodding. I feel cool. My heart isn't racing. . . . I don't have to go first at reporting. Someone else can start.

THERAPIST: How do you feel, and can you rate it?

SAMEENA: Calm and hopeful, 80%.

THERAPIST: How vivid is the antidote?

SAMEENA: Crystal clear.

THERAPIST: Is there anything else you need to help you feel calm and hopeful?

SAMEENA: No . . . that feels good.

THERAPIST: Well done. Let's have a quick rest and then try that again!

As before, the therapist(s) and client can monitor progress across successive practices, using the same chart (Appendix 8) as the one for practicing antidote image generation.

Once the client is able to swap the images in session, he or she is asked to practice this at home daily. Once a day, the client should bring to mind the old image; wait until he or she feels the toxic emotions (as before, up to about 70% intensity, but no more); and then swap in the antidote. As with assigning other types of homework, it may be helpful to negotiate when and where the client will do this practice (as well as to try to predict any obstacles). The client's experiences with this practice can then be discussed in session the following week.

The process of bringing the old image to mind and swapping in the antidote is a precursor to being able to swap in the antidote image spontaneously in everyday life, when the troubling image arises. The more the client practices doing this routinely, the more likely the client is to be able to do it spontaneously as needed. (Of course, in our experience, the rescripting of the troublesome image tends to result in its coming to mind less often anyway. So the need for such spontaneous image swapping decreases in most cases.)

The therapist(s) and client can "scaffold" image-swapping practice and spontaneous swapping with photographs, drawings, postcards, collage, computer graphics, sculptures, smells—whatever the client thinks will work. These personalized reminders can be placed around the client's home in conspicuous places, to prompt the client to practice.

CASE EXAMPLE: SAMEENA

Figure 9.7 shows Sameena's completion of a modified Microformulation Template (as usual, see Appendix 4 for a blank version), developed to describe the etiology and maintenance of an imagery "flashforward" of her performing badly at work meetings. As discussed throughout this chapter, Sameena appraised the image as meaning that she would definitely fail in her career. This led to her feeling utterly despairing and anxious. To cope with these unpleasant feelings, she resolved to avoid meetings and similar situations. However, this had the disadvantage of meaning that she *was* more likely to fail in her career; this would have created a vicious circle, whereby her avoidance made the intrusive imagery more likely to return. The therapist and Sameena worked to break this unhelpful cycle by

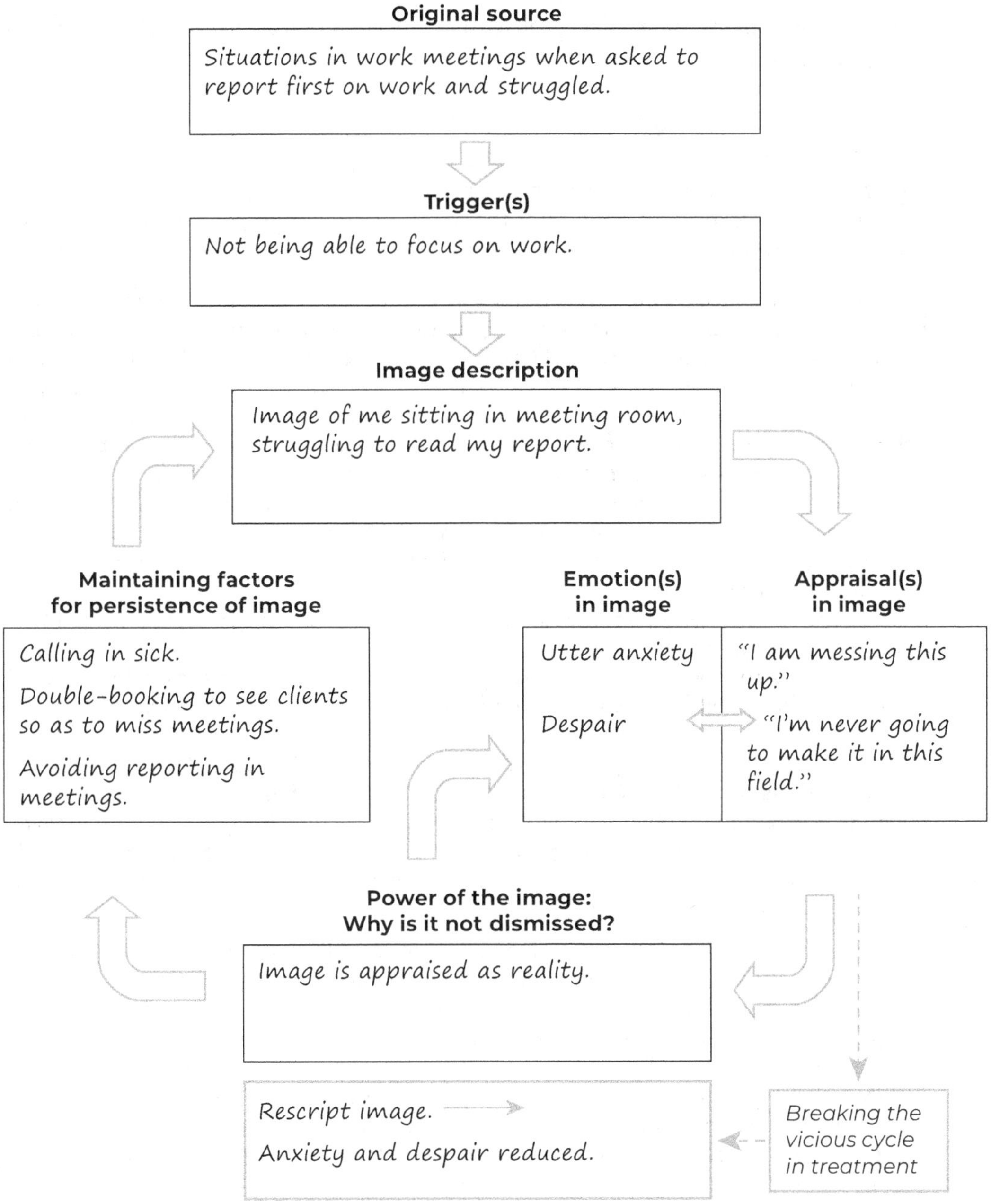

Original source

Situations in work meetings when asked to
report first on work and struggled.

Trigger(s)

Not being able to focus on work.

Image description

Image of me sitting in meeting room,
struggling to read my report.

**Maintaining factors
for persistence of image**

Calling in sick.

Double-booking to see clients
so as to miss meetings.

Avoiding reporting in
meetings.

**Emotion(s)
in image**

Utter anxiety

Despair

**Appraisal(s)
in image**

"I am messing this
up."

"I'm never going
to make it in this
field."

**Power of the image:
Why is it not dismissed?**

Image is appraised as reality.

Rescript image.
Anxiety and despair reduced.

Breaking the
vicious cycle
in treatment

FIGURE 9.7. Sameena's filled-in Microformulation Template (Appendix 4, somewhat modified/
streamlined for illustrative purposes), describing the etiology and maintenance of Sameena's target disruptive imagery. A potential "escape route" or way to break the cycle of intrusive imagery is indicated via
imagery rescripting.

rescripting the toxic image and replacing it with an antidote image that made her feel calm and hopeful—and, crucially, not needing to avoid meetings.

Hints and Tips for Imagery Rescripting

Here are three further considerations that may prove helpful in imagery rescripting.

First, if the client expresses doubt that the imagery rescripting procedure will be useful because the rescripted image "is not real," then the following explanation can be useful:

> "Athletes routinely use imagery techniques as part of their training routines. For example, Tom Daley, the British Olympic diver [or insert another appropriate figure, such as David Beckham, Carli Lloyd, Michael Phelps, or Katie Ledecky], has talked in the media about how he imagines himself doing a perfect dive over and over in his mind as a way of improving his performance in competitions. In reality, he may not ever be able to achieve the 'perfect' dive, as to be 100% perfect at anything is nearly impossible. However, when he comes to compete in an event, this mental imagery preparation helps him to perform well in real life. Many other athletes have noticed the same thing. What do you think would happen if instead Tom imagined himself messing up his dive over and over again? Do you think that this would be helpful in improving his performance? [At this point, most clients will agree that this is not helpful.]
>
> "So we can think of imagery rescripting as a way of finding an image for you that is more helpful for your life and your goals than the one that is currently causing you trouble. It does not need to be 100% 'real' or 'true'; it just needs to be something that will help you get on with the things you want to do in life, rather than hinder you."

Please also refer to the "Psychoeducation for Clients" section of Chapter 7, which includes further explanations about the effects of imagery on emotion, physiology, and behavior.

Second, "affect shift" (a change in emotion that can be indicated by a change in voice tone or posture, or by the client's own report) is the signal that the imagery rescripting is working. If the imagery rescripting procedure is not resulting in a change in affect, the following points may be useful to consider:

- Have all of the emotions and meanings associated with an image been elicited? One image can have more than one emotion and meaning attached to it, and these may be contradictory. It can be helpful to go back to the Chart for Constructing an Antidote for a Troublesome Image (Appendix 7) and see if any emotions or meanings have been omitted.
- If the image to be rescripted feels very threatening or distressing to the client (e.g., a memory of childhood trauma, or an image of suicide or self-harm), it may be necessary to create a safe or calming image first—one that the client can bring to mind to help decrease emotional arousal.
- Is the client holding back because the image still feels too powerful? Do the therapist(s) and client need to discuss the image and its power more?

Third, a client who struggles to describe a visual antidote image can try focusing on the bodily sensations in the troublesome image and then (with therapist help) generate an antidote to these. A visual antidote image can then be built up around the antidote sensations. As the client focuses on feeling these antidote sensations, does any image spring to mind? The therapist(s) should encourage the client to take some time for this; lots of images may come to mind, but one will present itself as the best option in the end.

CLIENT REFLECTIONS ON IMAGERY RESCRIPTING TECHNIQUES

The following are quotes from MAPP clients who were asked for feedback at the end of treatment. They reflect the usefulness of the imagery rescripting techniques these clients had learned to use.

"By the end of the process, not only was I able to engage with my 'imagery' thoughts, but I learned to interact with them and change them for the better."

"During the therapy, we went over the more upsetting side of the memories. They were like scenes from a movie, and I couldn't stop replaying them as a short video over and over, especially when I was anxious or stressed . . . and even worse, it was like the video got stuck on the most traumatic few seconds of the episode again and again. Each time I viewed the scene in my mind's eye, the same emotions came back—humiliation, sadness, fear—just as strongly as when it had happened for real. I hadn't recalled the memory on purpose, but I couldn't rid my mind of it. And there came back every detail—from where we were sitting, to . . . the scowl on her face, the tone of her voice, even the scents in the room. I couldn't change the scene or get rid of it . . . until I learned the MAPP techniques."

"I feel like I have been given the ultimate tool to help me manage my bipolar symptoms. I am now more in control of my mood swings because I can engage with my 'imagey' thoughts and change them for the better. Who even knew this was possible?"

CONCLUDING COMMENTS

In this chapter, we have described how to go through the five steps of imagery rescripting. We have shown that imagery rescripting is intended to change how clients *feel about* and *react to* a troublesome image. How this change is achieved, and how the image itself is transformed, are not important, as long as the rescripting changes how the client feels and reacts. Although imagery rescripting may seem quite cumbersome to begin with, therapists will find that clients get the "gist" of the technique very rapidly. As such, they are often able to rescript subsequent troubling images with very little help from their therapists. Imagery rescripting is often considered by therapists and clients alike to be the ultimate tool for dealing with intrusive imagery; it certainly seems the most powerful at times.

If a client's imagery problem is not one of negative images, but rather the problem of a paucity of more positive images, then a therapist may need to consider helping the client to generate such images. In the next chapter, we describe how to generate positive images.

CHAPTER 10

Promoting Positive Imagery

In MAPP, we define "positive imagery" as any mental imagery that holds a helpful and functional meaning for the individual experiencing it. The content of the image is in some ways unimportant; what matter are the *emotion* and *meaning* attached to it. Positive imagery may induce a sense of well-being, act to bolster self-esteem, or encourage the client to move in the direction of desired goals. It can be developed either by modifying existing unhelpful images; via imagery rescripting; or by creating new, "stand-alone" positive images. We focus on the last of these in this chapter.

The aim of this set of imagery techniques is to help clients to generate and practice positive images that can be used for a specific purpose. In MAPP, we have tended to use positive imagery interventions in two ways:

1. *As general strategies for inducing positive mood.* This approach is typically used, for example, when a client has a limited repertoire of positive experiences and positive past memories to draw upon. This can impede his or her ability to remain hopeful during treatment. The client may then be unable to engage fully with treatment, with the result that gains are not maintained over time. If we focus on generating a positive self-image (or future self-image) early in treatment, this can form a base on which to build other interventions. For example, we might help a client who was feeling very hopeless about his or her future to build and practice an image of what the client would hope to be feeling and doing in 1 year. If practiced daily, this positive, future-related image will act as a compelling goal to work toward in therapy. The daily practice will also engender regular feelings of hope.

Alternatively, a client may never have learned how to manage stressful situations or to regulate his or her own emotions. Positive imagery can be used as an effective calming and self-regulating strategy, to reduce distress and anxiety. "Safe place" imagery is particularly useful in these situations. (A detailed description of safe place imagery techniques is beyond the scope of this chapter. See Lee & James, 2012, for detailed information on how to use them.)

2. *As ways to address specific troublesome images.* As discussed in regard to imagery rescripting in Chapter 9, we can simply substitute a positive image for a troublesome one,

rather than going through the procedure of rescripting the troublesome image. Generally, we would choose this approach when there are too many troublesome images to rescript each individually, or because the troublesome images do not contain enough explicit information for rescripting. This can happen with, for example, memories from childhood that have few contextual details but strong emotional content.

A NOTE ABOUT POSITIVE IMAGERY IN THE CONTEXT OF BD

BD encompasses difficulties with elevated mood, and given that imagery can drive changes in mood and behavior, clinicians may understandably feel cautious about the use of positive imagery interventions with this population. It has been shown, for example, that people with BD experience positive future-related imagery as more vivid, exciting, and pleasurable than people with unipolar depression do (Ivins et al., 2014). Also, more pleasurable images are associated with higher scores on measures of drive and responsiveness to reward. In our experience, people with BD often spontaneously use positive imagery to encourage themselves to achieve targets (e.g., imagining receiving applause for a debut novel) or to generate a sense of being successful or popular (e.g., imagining others responding extremely positively to them in a social situation). However, they may not be fully aware of the potential for such images and their associated emotions to sustain and amplify feelings of elation or excitement. Creating and practicing imagery that involves ambitious goals, extreme achievement, or special recognition may not be functional for people with BD, even if they are in keeping with these individuals' abilities and desires. With this population, it is more helpful to work toward generating positive imagery linked to feelings of contentment, balance, and security, or imagery conveying a sense of being cared for. Such a focus also fits with the self-compassionate stance at the heart of the MAPP therapeutic ethos. We suggest that therapists discuss this issue openly with any clients with BD who are wanting to generate positive images containing extreme achievement.

RATIONALE FOR POSITIVE IMAGERY

In MAPP, we introduce the rationale of the positive mental imagery intervention by saying something like the following:

"As we have already discussed, mental images can have a powerful effect on emotions in both negative and positive ways. We can therefore harness the power of imagery to improve our mood. For instance, you might find yourself in a situation where you don't have the time or energy to challenge your emotions and thoughts, or find that reflecting on a problem actually makes you feel worse. Instead, what could be helpful in the here and now is a tool to help you improve your mood quickly, or to help you refocus on something different, or simply to give yourself a break. This is when positive imagery can be really helpful. It may sound odd and artificial to generate positive images in your mind, or you may be confused as to how this might work for you. However, as we have discussed before, our brains make no distinction between whether we are seeing some-thing in the mind's eye or perceiving it in the outside world—it is processed as if it were real. This means that it influences emotion and behavior just as powerfully as if it were really happening. Does that make sense? So, if you would like to try, we can generate some positive images that are relevant to you, and then we can test whether bringing those images to mind helps you feel more motivated, hopeful, relaxed, or whatever it is you have decided you need to feel. What do you think?"

DESCRIPTION OF STEPS

There are three basic steps to promoting positive imagery:

1. Agree on the rationale for using positive imagery (i.e., why is a positive image needed, or for what could it be helpful?).
2. Generate and test a positive image or images in session.
3. Make a plan for how the image(s) will be practiced in the client's everyday life.

Step 1: Agree on the Rationale for Using Positive Imagery

Using the shared microformulation as a guide, the therapist(s) and client should explore together in detail when, where, and with what aim the positive imagery will be used. This includes identifying the specifics of the situation with its emotional, cognitive, and behav-ioral components. Questions might include these:

- What is the problem to be addressed?
- How does the client feel? What does the client think and do?

Throughout this chapter, we discuss the example of Vivienne, a young mother who had previously worked as an environmental consultant. She experienced intrusive "flashfor-wards" to social occasions in which others would ask her what she had been doing recently. Vivienne saw a variety of images in which others looked awkward and their faces expressed pity and puzzlement when she would tell them that she had "just been at home." The images made her feel scared, disgusted, and ashamed. Because Vivienne experienced many differ-ent intrusive images, she and her therapist decided that using stand-alone positive imagery was more sensible than trying to rescript numerous images.

To return to the rationale for positive imagery, the problems to be addressed for Vivi-enne were the "flashforward" images that made her feel scared, disgusted, and ashamed, and that also led her to avoid social situations.

Once the client and therapist(s) are sure about the rationale for using positive imagery, the next step is for them to decide how the client ideally would *like to feel* (instead of how the client currently feels when he or she gets the images) and how the client would *like to behave* (instead of how he or she currently behaves). For instance, Vivienne said that she wanted to feel contented (rather than scared, disgusted, and ashamed), and that she would like to stop avoiding social situations.

In summary, then, the rationale for Vivienne was to generate a positive image that would help her feel contentment and stop her avoidance of social situations.

Step 2: Generate and Test Positive Image or Images in Session

The therapist(s) can start by guiding the client to remember the last time the client experienced an emotion similar to or matching the one he or she is aiming for (in Vivienne's case, the last time she felt contented). This can be at any time in the client's life, even in the very distant past. Based on knowledge of the client's personal history, the therapist(s) can, if appropriate, suggest situations, people, or places that might have been or still are related to the specific emotional meaning that is being sought. Alternatively, any image depicting the emotion that comes to mind for the client can be used (e.g., for Vivienne, this could have been a cartoon representing contentment, or a photograph of the sea).

If a client is struggling to generate positive images cued by specific people or memories, no one should worry; there are a number of other possibilities to explore (see the "Hints and Tips . . ." box at the end of this chapter). Therapists should avoid trying to make their own suggestions too quickly; allowing some quiet space often encourages an image to surface. We find that if a client sits with an emotion in mind for a few minutes, various mental images will present themselves, and after a while one will emerge as the "leader"—the one that the client would like to try out.

Once an initial image has been identified, the next step is to elaborate on it and rehearse it "live" in session. A therapist will first explain the procedure as described below, to make sure the client feels comfortable with each part of it.

Generating the Image

A therapist first instructs the client to bring the image to mind, and then asks the client to describe the image in as much detail as possible. Gentle prompts can be given to help the client elaborate on multisensory elements of the image (e.g., "What does it smell like?", "Can you feel anything in your body?"), to make it as rich and vivid as possible. The therapist can also remind the client, "Try to see the image through your own eyes and immerse yourself in it as much as possible." The client should be encouraged to generate the image with eyes closed, if possible.

Attaching Emotion

The therapist asks what emotion is being evoked by the image, and then asks the client to rate it on a scale of 0–100% (where 0% represents no emotion and 100% the most intense emotion the client has ever experienced). We advise aiming for a rating of 70–80%. If the emotional intensity is too low, the therapist can ask the client to try manipulating the image further (e.g., by asking, "What would you need to see, hear, or sense in the image to feel more like . . . ? Can you tune up the image—for example, make the colors brighter, or change anything else that could make the emotion more intense?"). If the emotion is too intense for the client, the therapist can also help to make it less so—for example, by asking the client to "turn down the volume" on the image in any way possible (this could include making it black and white, or imagining it at a distance). An example of "turning down" the emotion in an image, by making it black and white, has been given in Sameena's case in Chapter 9.

Checking That the Image Meets Its Aims

The therapist checks how the image makes the client *feel*, based on the client's direct feedback, on his or her emotional ratings, and also on nonverbal signals. (Observations of body language are important; if the aim of an the image is to promote a sense of calmness, for example, then the client will often spontaneously adopt a more relaxed posture.) The therapist also checks whether the generated image meets its aim in terms of *cognitions and behavior.* This is done by asking, "As you hold this image in your mind and as you are feeling X, what does that mean to you? What does it make you want to do?"

Feedback on Procedure

Once the client and therapists are satisfied with the live rehearsal of the positive image, then they should stop and debrief. It is important to gather information on challenges that occurred in the rehearsal session (e.g., the presence of unexpected emotions or distracting thoughts), in addition to what went well. This information will be used to modify the procedure if necessary.

Linking to a Cue

Once everyone is relatively happy with the image, it is also useful to discuss whether it could be associated with a smell (e.g., of a particular flower, fruit, essential oil, or perfume). We find that if clients practice associating the positive imagery with a smell, then over time, the smell can cue the image quite quickly. Other cues can also be useful, such as a picture or photograph that reminds a client of the positive image. If the client always looks at the picture or photograph when beginning to practice with the positive image, then, again, it will serve as a useful cue in the future.

It is generally a good idea to audio-record this exercise, so that the client can take away a recording of the image generation to help with possible difficulty in doing it at home alone. Listening to the recording may help cue the positive image. While most clients do not need the recording, it is worth making it anyway, just in case it is needed.

To demonstrate the technique of generating positive imagery, here is an excerpt from the therapy session in which Vivienne's positive image was generated.

> THERAPIST: Viv, are you happy with the procedure that I have just explained, for how we will try and generate the positive image?
>
> VIVIENNE: Yes, it sounds straightforward . . . um . . . but I am a little worried about whether or not it will work.
>
> THERAPIST: I understand that, and most people are worried before we get going. I know it sounds a bit strange. If it helps, I have yet to find someone who hasn't been

able to come up with a useful image . . . the mind always tends to present something. As we have discussed before, the good and bad news is that you are a high imager. The bad news is that you have vivid negative images . . . but the good news is that when you generate positive images, they too should be vivid and strong.

VIVIENNE: Yes, of course, that makes sense . . . let's do it!

THERAPIST: To remind you, we want to generate an image that makes you feel contentment and that makes you not want to avoid social situations. Let's start with that feeling of contentment. Can you think about a time recently, or not so recently, when you felt a strong sense of contentment? Take your time, there is no rush . . . just see what springs to mind.

VIVIENNE: Hmm . . . (*Thinks for a minute or two.*) It was last Easter. We had had a good day, and I was sitting with the kids in the conservatory [a solarium or sun room, for U.S. readers], and we were painting Easter eggs for them to take to the school fair. . . . You know, the kids had dipped their fingers in paint and were coloring the eggs like that. It was good fun, and I was proud of myself for doing this lovely creative thing with them, and I did feel contentment.

THERAPIST: Let's try that one, then. We can have a try at generating an image of that scene and see if it produces the positive emotions we want. If it doesn't, we will have a clearer idea of what we need by the end of it . . . so let's just give it a go.

[Note that this curious and experimental stance is important in imagery work. It takes the pressure off both therapist and client, and, crucially, allows the client to relax as much as possible, which means that his or her mind is free to be as creative as possible.]

THERAPIST: Can you close your eyes and focus on the day, last Easter, when you were sitting in the conservatory and you had been painting eggs? Can you tell me what is happening?

VIVIENNE: It was late afternoon. I was sitting in the conservatory at the table with the kids. Ben was on my left, and Alma was on my right.

THERAPIST: Can you describe what you can see around you, what the kids are wearing, how they look, and so on?

VIVIENNE: I can see the garden behind the conservatory windows. The cherry tree is starting to blossom . . . tiny white flowers. . . . The cat is purring on a chair in the corner, and the kids have their fingers all blue and yellow—they dip the fingers in the paint jars and then smudge the eggs—then Ben draws something blue on his sister's cheek . . . she giggles. The kids are both in denim shorts and t-shirts—matching. I said, "Snap—you look like identical twins!" when they came down to breakfast.

THERAPIST: Tell me more. What can you hear or smell?

VIVIENNE: Hmm . . . oh, birds chirping outside and the cat purring . . . and the kids giggling. Smell? The smell of wet paint—which I love.

THERAPIST: How does your body feel?

VIVIENNE: Warm and calm . . . the late afternoon sun is streaming in through the window and door. I can see the dust dancing in the sunlight around the blossom tree . . . you know how it does.

THERAPIST: Just concentrate on the image, on all the things around you in the conservatory, on that feeling in your body. What emotion do you feel, and how strong is it out of 100%?

VIVIENNE: I do feel contented . . . but . . . umm . . . only about 40% out of 100%, maybe.

THERAPIST: OK, what else do you need to feel contented? What else or who else do you need in the image for you to feel that feeling more strongly?

VIVIENNE: Hmm . . . (*Thinks for a minute.*) Maybe I need my partner to come downstairs . . . yes . . . and see what a lovely time we are having.

THERAPIST: OK, try that. Tell me what happens.

VIVIENNE: He runs down the stairs from his study . . . it's on the left . . . and walks into the conservatory. I hadn't heard his steps . . . he is wearing a checkered shirt and dark jeans like when he works from home, and he is smiling. It's Easter Monday . . . his eyes take in what we are doing, and he smiles . . . I love it when he smiles. His face crinkles up and his eyes shine . . . and he walks around to me, puts his hands on my shoulders, and says, "What have you guys been doing with your wonderful mummy?"

THERAPIST: How are you feeling as he says that?

VIVIENNE: Contentment and pride in myself—a good 90% out of 100%!

THERAPIST: Brilliant! And do you know, as you said that, your whole posture changed . . . you sat up straighter and took a big deep breath! So it looks like we have found a good image. Just keep it in mind for a minute for me, and focus on that lovely feeling of contentment—do you still feel it?

VIVIENNE: Yes, still strong.

THERAPIST: At this moment, as you feel like this . . . proud and contented . . . how do you feel about going to that social event next week?

VIVIENNE: Yeah. OK (*nodding and smiling*). I am a good mum, I am doing a good job, and that's what's important!

THERAPIST: Fantastic! Stay with that lovely feeling for a bit. Open your eyes when you are ready, and we can have a debrief and think about what smell or other cue it might be helpful to attach to the image.

Vivienne and the therapist discussed how the session had gone, and they agreed that both of them were happy with the positive image. They discussed what cue to try associating with the image. Candidates for the cue were the smell of wet paint (which reminded her of her kids), her partner's aftershave, and the smell of her blossoming tree. However, in the end, Vivienne decided that a photograph of the children (taken that Easter) would probably be most effective at cueing the positive image.

Step 3: Make a Plan for How the Image(s) Will Be Practiced in the Client's Everyday Life

Based on how the positive imagery generation has gone in session, the client and therapist(s) decide on how best it could be done as homework between sessions. As in any setting of CBT home practice, potential obstacles and ways to solve them are discussed, and a plan is jointly agreed upon. In our experience (and that of others), the practice of positive imagery between sessions is a crucial part of the intervention, allowing clients to scaffold and incorporate the technique into their everyday lives. It may be useful to offer the following explanation of the importance of home practice:

> "Imagery techniques are most effective when they are practiced on a daily basis. You can think of it as taking your daily medicine. If you had diabetes, you would take a daily dose of insulin. You need to take a daily dose of positive imagery for it to help you to feel better. Sometimes people find it hard to remember to take their medication, though, and this is quite normal. Let's think together about how we can help you remember to practice."

It is a good idea to make a home practice plan that includes a specific time and place to practice generating the positive imagery. At first it is helpful to practice in a situation where the client does not feel too emotionally aroused, where interruptions are unlikely, and where the client feels safe. For example, Vivienne decided to practice while she made her first cup of coffee in the morning. When the client has gained confidence in doing this, he or she can move on to bringing the positive imagery to mind in situations where the target difficulty is triggered.

The client should also be reminded to use the cue discussed in the session. If it is a smell, then the client should be encouraged to sniff it at the beginning of imagery home practice and at regular intervals throughout. If visual cues are used, the client should look at them at the beginning and end of the home practice (and in between if the client is struggling to generate a vivid image).

As mentioned earlier, clients may also like to listen to an audio recording of the imagery generation exercise that they did in the session, to help to remind them of the image.

If the positive imagery is being used to substitute for troubling images (as in Vivienne's case), then the client may need to practice this substitution in the session as well as for homework, as described in Chapter 9. This practice can be recorded on the Chart for Monitoring Progress in Practicing a Positive Image (see Appendix 9). For example, Vivienne practiced in session her bringing to mind a selection of recent negative images (in which she felt judged by others) and then substituting the positive imagery (of her in the conservatory with her children). Once she had done this successfully in the session, for homework she practiced the same exercise over the next week. Her filled-in chart, monitoring her progress over the week's practice, is shown in Figure 10.1. When Vivienne felt comfortable with this exercise, she moved on to substituting the positive for the negative images as they arose in her everyday life. With Vivienne, as with many other clients, we found that the negative images came much less frequently once they were either rescripted or replaced by positive images.

Write a brief description of the positive image, and then rate (on a scale of 0–100%) the intensity of the target emotions generated as you practice the image. Also rate how vivid the image is, on the same scale.

Positive Image	Target Positive Emotions and Vividness of Image Rate intensity of target emotions and vividness of image: 0–100%.						
	Practice 1	Practice 2	Practice 3	Practice 4	Practice 5	Practice 6	Practice 7
Me sitting in the conservatory with the children.	Content. Intensity: 70% Vividness: 70%	Content. Intensity: 70% Vividness: 80%	Content. Intensity: 80% Vividness: 80%	Content. Intensity: 60% Vividness: 70%	Content. Intensity: 80% Vividness: 80%	Content. Intensity: 85% Vividness: 90%	Content. Intensity: 85% Vividness: 80%

FIGURE 10.1. Vivienne's filled-in Chart for Monitoring Progress in Practicing a Positive Image (Appendix 9)

CASE EXAMPLES

Example 1: Vivienne

Vivienne was a young woman who was a stay-at-home mother for her two children, ages 3 and 6 years. Although she was a university graduate and had gone on to complete a master's degree in environmental science, she had found looking for paid employment after her first pregnancy too stressful, and elected to remain working in the home. Her partner ran his own business and often worked from home, which meant that they also had more time to see each other. Perhaps at some point she would join his business and work there too. Alongside a diagnosis of BD, Vivienne also presented with extreme social anxiety, which was triggered by images of others asking her in conversation what she had been doing lately. In the image, the question was followed by an awkward pause, and Vivienne saw their faces expressing pity and puzzlement. Vivienne experienced this intrusive image whenever there was a forthcoming social event. It made her feel scared and disgusted, and made her think that others saw her as living a wasteful life. She also reported a sense of shame, and the thought that she was "using resources on the planet without contributing" made her feel depressed. The image was very vivid and real, with multisensory elements: She could feel herself blushing and sweating in the image, and her stomach churning. Vivienne could not stop herself from going over and over these images in her mind, with the result that she was beginning to avoid all social situations.

Vivienne and her therapists agreed that it could be helpful to generate positive images of herself to break this vicious cycle. In fact, Vivienne was proud of the way she took care of her children—stimulating their interests and abilities by always organizing creative activities for them and taking them to different places. She also acknowledged that everyone praised her for being a very good host and friend. Her partner was particularly grateful and loving, and valued her advice on his own business.

In session, as described above, Vivienne rehearsed an image where she viewed herself though her own eyes sitting in the conservatory painting Easter eggs with her children, and then her partner came in to join them. The image conveyed a feeling of contentment at being at the center of her family. At first, Vivienne practiced this image when she had some quiet moments to herself during the day. She then moved on to rehearsing them prior to attending social situations. She noticed that this made the negative image intrude less frequently, and that it became less vivid and intense.

Figure 10.2 shows Vivienne's modified Microformulation Template (as usual, see Appendix 4 for a more complete blank version of this form), developed to describe the etiology and maintenance of her target disruptive imagery. A potential way to break the cycle of intrusive imagery is indicated via use of positive imagery.

Example 2: Batinder

Batinder was a young student who had been recently diagnosed with BD. He had needed to repeat a year of university due to a combination of recurrent depressive episodes and hypomanic states, triggered at the times of exams. Although he was not currently depressed, minor mishaps during his seminars were easily perceived as signs that he would fail again.

Original source

Social events shortly after left paid work.

Trigger(s)

Forthcoming dinner parties.

Partner talking about social occasion.

Image description

Conversations between myself and other people, viewed through their eyes. Being asked what I have been doing lately, and there is a pause. I then see their faces, which show pity and puzzlement.

Maintaining factors for persistence of image	**Emotion(s) in image**	**Appraisal(s) in image**
Go over and over image in mind, imagining all possible scenarios. Avoid social situations.	Fear Disgust Shame Depression	"Other people think I am wasteful." "Other people pity me." "I should be doing more to help the planet." "I'm using up precious resources without contributing."

Power of the image: Why is it not ignored?

Image is appraised as reality.

Image is highly vivid and detailed and has multisensory elements: very compelling

Generate and rehearse (1) images of positive roles (e.g., in the family) and achievements, (2) images that promote calmness and confidence.

Breaking the vicious cycle in treatment

FIGURE 10.2. Vivienne's filled-in Microformulation Template (Appendix 4, somewhat modified/streamlined for illustrative purposes), describing the etiology and maintenance of Vivienne's target disruptive imagery. A potential "escape route" or way to break the cycle of intrusive imagery is indicated via use of positive imagery.

These could then lead to his feeling stuck, unable to get out of bed to attend any class or to go to the library. When asked about these situations, he was not able to identify any particular thought or emotion other than lying in bed with "my mind blank, my body stuck, I just don't have the energy." When eventually some external trigger (such as a friend picking him up to go for their swimming training together) dragged Batinder out of bed, he could easily get back into his normal routine. However, if this did not happen by chance, his mood could become quickly depressed, as he was unable to motivate himself to do the activities that would help him feel better.

In a MAPP session, Batinder agreed to try bringing to mind a positive image that could make him feel energized enough to get started in the day. Batinder reported that on mornings when he felt good, his limbs didn't feel so heavy, and he could focus on the places he needed to get to (a seminar, the library, the university pool). He summed up his goal as feeling "light, energized, and focused." He would need to be able to generate an image on his own when he was lying in the dark of his bedroom and his housemates had already left for the day.

Batinder remembered that he used to feel energized and light as a child when he went to swimming competitions on weekend mornings. He disliked getting up, but liked going with other children in a minivan and having "special" chocolate bars prior to a race. Using this memory as a cue in session, Batinder generated an image where he could see the light blue swimming pool surface gently undulating in front of him and smell the chlorine. Initially this image conveyed a sense of lightness and excitement, but also some anxiety. In order to maintain only the energizing part of the feeling, Batinder decided to add the sound of children's chatter and the sensation after the race of putting on his soft bathrobe after getting out of the water. This way, the image incorporated lightness and energy, but not the precompetitive rush of adrenaline and anxiety. While generating the image, he would sit more upright and with his chest more open; holding the image in mind made him feel much more like wanting to go out and get on with life.

At the next therapy session, Batinder reported that he had tried practicing the positive image two or three times. On one occasion, he was only able to bring the image of the pool to mind for a few seconds and could not reproduce the rest of the sensations associated with it. The therapist encouraged him to describe what else had happened, and he realized that as soon as he had brought his positive image to mind, he had also started questioning it. For example, he thought, "This is silly; it doesn't make any sense," and "I never won any competition, so those swimming races were not so nice in reality." Both Batinder and his therapist noticed that the positive image was missing one of the emotions that he wanted it to have: the sense of being "focused." Interestingly, the therapist wondered whether being focused could also help prevent him from ruminating about the positive image. Batinder described "focused" as the sensation he associated with physical challenge and perhaps a sense of muscular exertion. The therapist encouraged him to try and integrate this into the positive image. Batinder then devised a second image where he imagined himself swimming through the water, with a rhythmic splashing sound and a mild sense of tension in his muscles that made him feel the sense of focus he had lacked in the previous image. Batinder found that this new image was useful in helping him get up in the morning and carry out his everyday tasks and studies.

Hints and Tips for Promoting Positive Imagery

If a client is unable to identify ideas for positive images, here are some suggestions for therapists:

- Encourage the client to brainstorm any pictures, music, sounds, smells, or objects that could theoretically trigger the desired emotion. These can be familiar and personal to the client; a fantasy image, such as the perfect beach; or a metaphorical image (e.g., calming waves, energizing sunshine, or steadfast mountains).
- Use materials such as postcards, fragrances, or plasticine/modeling clay, which can help to calm and ground the client.
- Explore positive roles (e.g., mother, father, teacher, friend) that the client plays in his or her life now, and use them as cues for the image.
- Have the client imagine developing a positive image not for him- or herself, but for someone the client trusts and cares for. What would the client want this person to imagine?

If a client is unable to bring to mind any positive image, therapists can remember the following:

- Images are multisensory, so a client can start developing an image with a nonvisual component.
- An emotion can be represented by a bodily feeling and can be a useful place to start from if a client (or a therapist) is feeling stuck. For example, a client who needs the positive image to help him or her feel calm can be asked what physical sensations are associated with a sense of calmness. These might include shoulders dropping, the breath becoming more relaxed, or the like. The therapist can help the client to focus on those physical sensations, and after a while, various visual images will come to the client's mind to "bulk out" the positive image (e.g., visualizing being fully suspended in water and observing beautiful fish passing by).
- Clients should be reminded that as imagery is all about imagination, there is no "right" or "wrong" image. In fact, trying out even an unsatisfactory image may open up the creative process that will eventually lead to a helpful one.
- Also, therapists need to remain calm and reassuring themselves. If a nervous client is told to relax and take as much time as necessary, eventually an image will come to mind.

If a client is generating positive imagery that is too extreme, therapists can do the following:

- Dedicate additional time to psychoeducation, and collaboratively formulate the potential pitfalls of overly positive imagery (e.g., images depicting perfection or ultimate success).
- Explore the effect of "balanced imagery" on mood and behavior—for example, images representing being "good enough," embracing both a client's strengths and weaknesses.

If a client does not want to close his or her eyes, therapists can keep these points in mind:

- Mental imagery will work better if clients close their eyes; this is simply because the external visual environment will act as a distractor.
- Nevertheless, some clients, particularly those with a history of trauma, may not wish to close their eyes. It is useful if therapists explore briefly what such clients fear may

happen if they close their eyes, and whether the therapists and clients can do anything together to help reduce the fear.

- Encourage these clients to try the exercise with eyes closed, with the proviso that the clients can open their eyes whenever they wish.
- Ultimately, if a client is too afraid to close his or her eyes and there is nothing that a therapist can do to reduce that fear, then the development of imagery will have to proceed with open eyes.

CLIENT REFLECTION ON USING POSITIVE IMAGERY

The following is a quote from a MAPP client who was asked for feedback at the end of treatment. It reflects the usefulness of the positive imagery that the client had learned to use.

"At the beginning you may think, 'Right, as if all the other symptoms weren't enough, now there's also this thing of having incredibly vivid mental images,' and you realize how scared or hopeless those images can make you feel. But at the end of MAPP, I figured out there was a silver lining and it was in my hands to twist this new 'images thing' around—because if you have super-vivid mental images, you can imagine something good and relaxing, and then you feel really positive or calm."

CONCLUDING COMMENTS

In this chapter, we have explained when and how to generate positive images with a client. As with other imagery techniques, the precise details of the images do not matter greatly, as long as they make the client *feel* the target positive emotions and want to *behave* in the target way. Positive images are clearly useful as a "stand-alone" method of inducing a better mood. They can also be used as substitutes for more negative images if imagery rescripting is not possible (e.g., if there are too many different kinds of negative images). In the next chapter, we explore the use of imagery-competing tasks; these too can be helpful when a client has lots of different troublesome images.

CHAPTER 11

Introducing
Imagery-Competing Tasks

One approach to managing distressing and intrusive images can be to disrupt them or reduce their impact by using competing visuospatial tasks. "Visuospatial tasks," as the term indicates, can be any tasks or activities that involve significant visual and spatial components. Common visuospatial activities in everyday life include playing a visual computer game, creating a painting or sculpture, playing a musical instrument, playing various sports (e.g., tennis or football), and doing a jigsaw puzzle.

This sort of activity can be used in MAPP therapy in two ways: (1) as a targeted intervention technique *within sessions* to reduce the impact and frequency of a distressing, intrusive image; and (2) as a general coping strategy to manage distressing images in day-to-day life, *outside of sessions.*

Using competing tasks to disrupt imagery can be useful when imagery rescripting is not felt to be appropriate as a first option. This might happen, for example, if a client and therapist(s) have not yet been able to explore the meaning of the images, but an immediate coping strategy is needed. Alternatively, it can be useful when a client is troubled by a high volume of different images. In this case, it would not be feasible to intervene in some way with each image; rather, a strategy that will help address *all* images is preferable.

Research in cognitive psychology suggests that visuospatial tasks can be used to disrupt distressing visual images and reduce their vividness, possibly by competing for visual processing resources. In simple terms, we suspect that the brain cannot attend equally to the distressing images *and* to the visuospatial task; thus the impact of the distressing images is diminished or diluted. Two threads of this research are of interest.

1. First, we know that visuospatial activities such as modeling in clay or playing the computer game Tetris have been found to reduce how often distressing images "intrude" (i.e., make an unbidden appearance) in daily life, when carried out soon after a distressing event. In the procedure that has been tested, there is a brief reminder cue to bring the image to mind, and then a person engages in a visuospatial activity for a sustained period— approximately 15 minutes (e.g., Iyadurai et al., 2018; Holmes et al., 2009). For older memories, the procedure requires "reactivating" the image (i.e., deliberately bringing the image to mind or having an intrusion of the image), followed by about a 10-minute wait before the

visuospatial task will be effective (e.g., James et al., 2015). Then a client needs to engage in the visuospatial task for approximately 15 minutes or more. Another option is for a client to do the visuospatial task continually after the memory reactivation for the full 25 minutes. Following from this research, we found that if our clients brought a target troublesome image to mind in MAPP and then (for instance) played Tetris for 20 minutes or more, the visuospatial activity helped to disrupt the image and reduce its rate of intrusion thereafter.

2. Second, we know from research that performing a visuospatial task at the same time as a distressing image is held in mind has been shown to reduce the vividness and emotional impact of the image as rated by nonclinical participants in the laboratory (Engelhard et al., 2010; Kavanagh et al., 2001), and even clients with PTSD (Lilley, Andrade, Turpin, Sabin-Farrell, & Holmes, 2009). We suspect that images that are less vivid and emotional feel less real and are easier to dismiss or detach oneself from. Following from this, we found that our MAPP clients were able to use visuospatial tasks outside of sessions as a general strategy for coping when distressing images occurred.

RATIONALE FOR IMAGERY-COMPETING TASKS

It is important to begin by explaining the technique and how it works to clients. This will help them to understand how and when to use it, and to decide whether or not to try it. A therapist can use this simple explanation:

"Certain activities can be used to disrupt upsetting images. The sorts of activities that work include ones that involve using visual and spatial skills. Common examples are art, modeling, playing a musical instrument, or playing a computer game such as Tetris. We think that these activities work because our brains can only process so much information in the same modality (or form) at one time. That is why, when you are talking to someone on the telephone (which is a verbal activity), you can *watch* what is happening on TV at the same time (which is a visual activity), but you cannot *listen* to what the person on TV is saying (which is a verbal activity). In other words, it is very difficult to do two verbal tasks at the same time. In the same way, when you are playing Tetris, which is a visual activity, it is difficult to hold another visual image in mind. In fact, research has shown that a therapy procedure including tasks like Tetris can make distressing images less vivid and emotional, and can reduce how often these images pop into mind from day to day."

DESCRIPTION OF STEPS

There are four steps for using a visuospatial task in session:

1. Identify the target image.
2. Reactivate (bring to mind) the target image and check that it is vivid (by rating it).
3. Carry out the visuospatial task.
4. Rerate the target image.

Step 1: Identify the Target Image

If the client is having a number of distressing images, the client and therapist(s) should identify one that is strongly visual and is currently having a notable impact on the client's life. For example, in the case of Zheng (described later in this chapter), one of her recurrent images of various scenarios of performing badly at university might be a suitable target.

Step 2: Reactivate the Target Image and Check That It Is Vivid

The client begins by closing his or her eyes and bringing the target image to mind. Then the client is asked to describe what the image is like and how it makes him or her feel, to check that the image is vivid, visual, and distressing. It may be helpful to take brief ratings of vividness and distress (e.g., on a 0–100% scale where 0% = not at all and 100% = extremely).

If the image is not vivid enough (the aim is a rating of 70% or more), the therapist(s) should work with the client to make it more vivid—for example, by asking for more details about all of the senses in the image ("What can you hear/feel in your body/smell?"); ensuring that the client is seeing it through his or her own eyes, not as an observer; suggesting that the client "turn up" the colors (or sounds, etc.); and making sure that the client isn't "holding back" from immersion in the image, due to fear. If fear is a problem, it will be sensible to explore the client's fears and seek ways to reassure him or her.

A practical note is that taking these ratings and working with the client to increase the vividness can help to fill up the 10-minute wait after image reactivation (see step 3, below)—a time period that is thought to be needed before the visuospatial task is likely to start taking effect.

Step 3: Carry Out the Visuospatial Task

Once 10 minutes have elapsed after the most recent reactivation of the image, the client should be asked to carry out the chosen visuospatial activity without interruption for at least 10 minutes, and preferably for 20 minutes or more. Any visuospatial activity can be used, as long as the client is willing to try it, and as long as it can be carried out feasibly within a session. As indicated previously, activities such as painting, modeling in clay, or playing visual computer games often work well. In our experience, the computer game Tetris (using Marathon mode) is particularly effective and easy to use. The game can be played on a computer (*https://tetris.com* or *www.tetrislive.com*), mobile phone, or hand-held gaming device. Sample instructions for explaining how to play Tetris, emphasizing the use of mental rotation, are given here.

> "Now I'm going to ask you to have a go at playing the computer game Tetris. Have you heard of the game before or played it? [Depending on the client's familiarity with the game, give either a brief explanation, or a fuller explanation with a demonstration as described below.]
>
> "The game consists of seven different-shaped blocks, which fall from the top of the screen one at a time. The aim of the game is to move and rotate the blocks to make complete horizontal lines across the screen. Each time you fill a whole line with the

blocks, the line will disappear, and the game will give you points. The aim is to fill as many lines as possible before the playing screen is filled up with blocks.

"In particular, I want you to focus on the block [in *www.tetrislive.com*]/blocks [in *https://tetris.com*] that will be falling immediately after the one being played, showing at the top right of the screen. Try to work out in your mind's eye how best to rotate and place the blocks in order, to fill the lines as efficiently as possible.

"You can move the blocks left and right by using the cursor keys here, and you can rotate them by 90° one way or the other, using these other cursor keys here. If you are confident that you have a block at the rotation and position you want, you can speed up how fast it falls by pressing the down key.

"Do you have any questions? Would you like to have a practice?" [If necessary, give the client an opportunity to practice the game, until the client is confident that he or she understands the instructions.]

Step 4: Rerate the Target Image

After the visuospatial activity, the client should bring the distressing image to mind and rate it again. This will help the therapist(s) and client to see if the activity has had an effect. The client should also be asked what he or she thought of the technique and whether it felt helpful.

If the client has found using a visuospatial task helpful in the session, the therapist(s) may suggest that the client try using the technique (Steps 1–4) on a day-to-day basis, whenever an intrusive or distressing image occurs.

It is important to identify one or more visuospatial activities that the client is willing to do regularly, that can be accessed easily (e.g., playing the piano may not be suitable when the client is at work), and that engage visuospatial processing sufficiently to disrupt the imagery. This may involve identifying a number of options in the session and asking the client to experiment with them at home to see what works best. If the client has found playing Tetris helpful in the session, two options might be for him or her to download the game onto a smartphone from *https://tetris.com* or to play it online at home.

It may also be helpful to ask the client to record the vividness and distress associated with the image(s) on the 0–100% scale before and after the visuospatial activity, just as he or she did in the session. This will give helpful information about whether the technique is effective. Appendix 10 is a blank form for recording this practice. Clients may also find it helpful to monitor the number of intrusive images they experience, say over one week, both before and after using the technique.

CASE EXAMPLES

Example 1: Zheng

Zheng was a 24-year-old university student with a 4-year diagnosis of BD Type II. She reported having lots of different intrusive images, most of which were "flashforward" images. Some of these images predicted poor performance at university; some predicted negative evaluation of her appearance by others; and some showed her placing herself in danger or harming herself. These images occurred many times a day and left her feeling "paralyzed with fear." On a number of occasions, the images had been so compelling that she had canceled or avoided appointments, and this pattern of avoidance had begun to affect her study performance and her friendships. Her Microformulation Template (Appendix 4, somewhat modified as usual for illustrative purposes) is shown in Figure 11.1.

In a MAPP treatment session, Zheng described a particularly distressing "flashforward" of an upcoming meeting with her supervisor. After bringing the image to mind in the session, and then rating the image and receiving instructions on playing Tetris while she and the therapist waited for the necessary time to elapse (see steps 2 and 3 above), she played the game for about 20 minutes. Immediately after this, Zheng found that when she tried to bring the image to mind again, it was harder to picture and felt less real. Before her next session, Zheng decided to download Tetris onto her phone and use it at night (within Steps 1–4) before she went to bed, when she tended to find it harder to dismiss the images; this helped her to get to sleep. After a few weeks, she reported fewer intrusive "flashforward" images of her university performance, and found that they felt less real, vivid, and compelling.

Example 2: Kofi

Kofi was a 43-year-old man who described repeated compelling images of his wife being in an accident. The content of the images varied from day to day, depending on what his wife was doing. For example, if his wife was on a work trip that day, he might see her seriously injured in a car accident. He found that he tended to dwell on the images, and often elaborated them in his mind (e.g., imagining himself going to a hospital and seeing his wife injured or dying). The images were extremely distressing, as he believed they meant that he was a bad husband. The images tended to occur once he got back home from work, if he was on his own before the rest of the family returned. Once his wife returned home, he felt that he was often overly anxious and asked her lots of questions about what had happened that day, which was irritating for her.

Kofi enjoyed playing keyboard instruments and imagining the music unfold before him. He found that if he played one of his keyboards in the evenings, it disrupted the images and prevented him from dwelling on them. After a while, he found that the images were no longer so compelling, and he realized that they did not predict what would happen. This meant that Kofi could feel more relaxed with his wife in the evenings.

Hints and Tips for Using Imagery-Competing Tasks

- Check that the image to be disrupted is predominantly visual. If it is mainly auditory, tactile, or olfactory, visuospatial tasks may not be as effective. If the image is predominantly auditory, the client and therapist(s) can experiment with disrupting it by using competing auditory tasks (e.g., singing along to music, counting, reciting the multiplication tables or poetry, reading aloud) within the Steps 1–4 procedure.
- Therapists should explore with clients what works for them. This may be to use a technique at particular times, when the clients know they tend to have distressing images (e.g., at night when they are trying to sleep, as in Zheng's case), or to experiment with different types of activities as the images arise during the day. Follow each of Steps 1–4.

Original source

> *Nothing could be identified.*

Trigger(s)

> *Upcoming university/social event (e.g., seminars, lunch with university friends).*

Image description

> (1) *Socially humiliating images (e.g., mind goes blank in class).*
> (2) *Negative images of body.*
> (3) *Images of putting self in dangerous situations on purpose (e.g., walking in parks alone at night).*
> (4) *Images of harming self.*

Maintaining factors for persistence of image

> *Elaborate on images (e.g., imagine further).*
>
> *Act on images (e.g., actually walk around parks at night, look things up online, or go shopping).*
>
> *Avoid activity (e.g., do not go to work).*
>
> *Images affect sleep and concentration.*

Emotion(s) in image	**Appraisal(s) in image**
Anxious	*"I'm going to fail."*
Humiliated	*"Everyone thinks I'm weird/odd/ugly."*
Depressed	*"This is what my future will be like. I don't deserve anything else."*

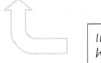

Power of the image: Why is it not dismissed?

> *Images are appraised as real and as having meaning.*

> *Disrupt images by using competing visual task (e.g., Tetris).*
>
> *Reduction in image vividness, realness, and "compellingness."*

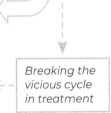

> *Breaking the vicious cycle in treatment*

FIGURE 11.1. Zheng's filled-in Microformulation Template (Appendix 4, somewhat modified/streamlined for illustrative purposes), describing the etiology and maintenance of Zheng's target disruptive imagery. A potential "escape route" or way to break the cycle of intrusive images is indicated via use of competing visuospatial tasks.

- Sometimes it is not possible for a client to do a visuospatial activity for as long as 20 minutes, because the client may wish to take a break part way through. However, before the client resumes the visuospatial activity after such a break, it is important to bring the original troubling image to mind again briefly (and then wait 10 minutes).

CLIENT REFLECTION ON USING IMAGERY-COMPETING TASKS

The following is a quote from a MAPP client who was asked for feedback at the end of treatment. It reflects the usefulness of using Tetris to disrupt unpleasant imagery, once such imagery had already intruded into the client's mind.

"Initially I wasn't sure about changing the images—I mean, about focusing on a really bad one and making it into something different—so the team suggested I try using Tetris as part of a 4-step procedure to interrupt the images from flooding in my mind. For me, the images would disturb me as I tried to get to sleep, but I need my sleep to keep things on track (it's one of the first things you learn about being bipolar). So I would feel upset by the images and then worried about not sleeping, and then just more and more helpless. Discovering there was something really simple to break this pattern was great. . . . It's not rocket science when you think about it, but it had never occurred to me. Now I tell everyone in my family to use this procedure and play Tetris when they are worrying about work stuff or about having to meet someone the next day!"

CONCLUDING COMMENTS

In this chapter, we have explained how to describe and implement an unusual but useful technique for disrupting and reducing the frequency of troublesome mental images: engaging in a competing visuospatial task. Once an image is brought to mind, it may be important to do the task uninterrupted and with sufficient duration for it to take effect. Using imagery-competing tasks is a relatively new way of dealing with troublesome images, but recent clinical research suggests that it can reduce the number of intrusive images when used soon after a traumatic event (e.g., Iyadurai et al., 2018), although further research is needed. Furthermore, dismantling studies (van den Hout & Engelhard, 2012) indicate that a similar process of competition for working memory resources explains the effectiveness of another imagery-based technique, eye movement desensitization and reprocessing (EMDR; see Shapiro, 2018), for PTSD. Whatever the precise mechanism, imagery-competing tasks are easy to use and portable; they give clients a tool they can quickly adopt in their everyday lives once troubling imagery arises. Remember, the task alone is not enough; use all four steps of the procedure.

We have now come to the end of the treatment techniques that we used within the MAPP case series. In the next chapter, we describe how we worked with clients to consolidate their learning.

CHAPTER 12

Consolidation Sessions
Making Video Blueprints

In the latter stages of MAPP treatment, two sessions are devoted to helping clients consolidate the gains they have made, and in particular the strategies they have learned to help them manage their emotions. Focusing explicitly on consolidation is important, because we want our clients to be able to cope with unexpected future events, without necessarily thinking that they need more therapy. We want them to have a summary in an accessible format of what they have learned, to consult if the need arises.

Thus the two broad aims of the two MAPP consolidation sessions are these:

1. Help the client to consolidate and embed the strategies learned over the course of the MAPP treatment sessions.
2. Create a record of these strategies that the client can return to in the future.

In traditional CBT, a paper-based "blueprint" is typically produced by the client and therapist at the end of therapy to summarize the learning that has taken place over the course of the CBT sessions and to document relapse prevention strategies. In the MAPP intervention, the client and therapist(s) depart from the traditional paper-based blueprint format and instead produce a "video blueprint"—that is, a visual record of the client's learning.

The idea for the use of video blueprints came from a study by Walton and Cohen (2011), which used a video-based social belonging intervention to improve health and academic outcomes for minority students. However, the rationale for using video blueprints in MAPP is multifaceted:

- As discussed earlier in this manual, people with BD may have a predisposition to be "visualizers" rather than "verbalizers." Therefore, tailoring CBT techniques to suit this style

135

of processing may enable clients with BD to use them more effectively. There is evidence from neuropsychological studies that visual memory may be less affected by BD than verbal memory may be.

  • More generally, there is evidence that we all have enhanced recall for situations that are novel and in which a moderate degree of stress is present. Most people in the general population would agree that having a film or video made of themselves is somewhat anxiety-provoking or stressful, and for most people it is not a day-to-day occurrence. Therefore, the use of a novel, moderately anxiety-provoking technique to produce a blueprint is again aimed at enhancing memory for the content of the blueprint.

  • There is evidence from research in social psychology that people are more likely to endorse messages that are freely advocated; this is called the "saying-is-believing" effect (e.g., Aronson, Fried, & Good, 2002). Therefore, videoing clients talking about, for example, the strategies that have helped them to improve their mood stability encourages them to internalize the message they are giving.

  • In the aforementioned study by Walton and Cohen (2011), minority students were asked to deliver a message to the camera, which they believed would be shown to new students, to "help ease their transition to college." The authors argued that this stance might avert any perceived stigma associated with receiving an intervention, as the participants were encouraged to see themselves "as benefactors and not as beneficiaries." What Walton and Cohen found was that the students who recorded the messages reported improved health and academic outcomes. When producing video blueprints in our MAPP case series, we asked clients to give a message to someone who might find themselves in a similar position, perhaps someone newly diagnosed with BD. We hoped this would help clients to see themselves as benefactors, with useful skills to share with others.

If therapists work in an environment where the use of sophisticated video equipment would be difficult (perhaps because of financial or space constraints), then lots of other options are possible: recording a video blueprint on a client's smartphone; recording the blueprint in audio format only; or drawing a diagram or picture to encapsulate the information in the blueprint. The important factor is to try to make the blueprint as memorable as possible, and to record it in a format that the client will easily be able to use if he or she is struggling in the future.

OVERVIEW OF THE TECHNIQUE

Clients are introduced to the idea and rationale behind the consolidation intervention at the end of the fourth and final session in the active treatment phase of MAPP. The main consolidation intervention, the production of the video blueprint, takes place in consolidation session 1. The clients and therapists then watch and discuss the video together in consolidation session 2, and a copy of the blueprint is given to the client to take home.

RATIONALE FOR A VIDEO BLUEPRINT

A therapist might explain the rationale for making a video blueprint to consolidate the intervention as follows:

"We have completed your active treatment sessions together now, and you have worked hard to learn and put in place a lot of useful strategies to help stabilize your mood. What we want to do now is to make sure that you remember these strategies and have a record of them for the future. Does that make sense?

[Client responds.]

"So what we are going to do in our next session may sound a little unusual, but we can reassure you that previous clients have told us that they found it helpful. Rather than write down the strategies you have learned on a piece of paper, what we are going to do is make a video together that you can keep and watch in the future. We call this a 'video blueprint.'

"We understand that most people feel a little self-conscious about the idea of making a video of themselves. So do we! However, this is actually one of the reasons we use this format: We know that people are better at remembering experiences that are a little out of the ordinary and a little anxiety-provoking. Therefore, we hope that making this video will really help to embed this learning in your memory. It is also a very image-based record, which people with BD may find easier to remember than written documents. Do you have any questions or immediate thoughts about this?

[Most people will say that they do not like the idea of making a film or video of themselves. A therapist can reassure such a client that this is entirely normal, can explore any fears about making a video, and can highlight common discrepancies between expectations and reality (e.g., about seeing/hearing oneself on a video).]

"There is no one way of doing the video blueprint. We can make a video of you talking to the camera, or of the two [or three, if there are cotherapists] of us having a conversation together. Or you might have another creative idea that you would like to use for the video—for example, making use of drawings or objects. Do you have any initial thoughts about that?

[A client who is very opposed to appearing in a video should not feel coerced into doing so. However, we recommend encouraging clients to be videoed if possible. If a client is strongly opposed to being videoed, then here are some other options: the cotherapists having a conversation on camera (with the client talking off camera); or the cotherapists talking on camera from a script written by the client; or videoing a piece of paper on which the client draws representations of the strategies he or she has learned, while describing them in detail.]

"What we'd like you to do before our next session is to consider this list of core guide questions, which will help you to think about the information that is important to include in the video blueprint. It would be great if you could note down any things you think would be particularly helpful to include for each of the questions. Please feel free to expand these questions and to include anything else that you think would be helpful. The video blueprint is a document for you to keep and refer back to, so you can tailor it in any way to suit you."

DESCRIPTION OF STEPS

There are six main steps involved in producing and reviewing a video blueprint:

1. Introduce the rationale and procedure for producing the video blueprint.
2. Give the client the list of core guide questions to consider.
3. Discuss the client's answers to the core guide questions and plan the video.
4. Produce the video blueprint.
5. Review and discuss the blueprint together in session.
6. Give the client a copy of the blueprint.

Step 1: Introduce the Rationale and Procedure for Producing the Video Blueprint

Following discussion of the rationale with the client (as described above), the therapist(s) will explain that the first part of the next session (consolidation session 1) will focus on reviewing and planning the information to be included in the video and planning the structure of the video. Then the main part of this session will be spent in making the video. The therapist(s) will also let the client know that in consolidation session 2, they will review the video together, and the client will be given a copy to take home with him or her.

Step 2: Give the Client the List of Core Guide Questions to Consider

The core guide questions are as follows. (Please note that the client can revise or add to these; they should not be seen as rigid requirements.)

- What did you learn in the MAPP sessions?
- What will you do to continue making good progress in the future?
- What will you do/need to remember to be kind to yourself in future?
- If you were having a "blip" in the future, what would you want to remind yourself of or say to yourself?
- Finally, if you were giving advice to someone in a similar position to yourself—perhaps someone newly diagnosed with BD—what message would you want to give this person, to help him or her feel that things were more manageable?

The therapist(s) should encourage the client to be playful and creative. There is no one way to do a video blueprint (see the box below for some examples).

Finally, the client should be instructed to begin thinking through the core guide questions, and perhaps making notes at home, in preparation for the next session.

Examples of Video Blueprints Produced by MAPP Clients

- A play in which three puppets (voiced by the client and two cotherapists) discussed imagery and what they had learned in MAPP.
- A beautiful tree in a park, with a voiceover saying, "An image is just an image."
- The client drawing the strategies with colored pens on a piece of paper, while talking them through.
- A three-way conversation among the two cotherapists and the client, in which the therapists asked questions from the consolidation list and the client answered them.
- A PowerPoint presentation made by the client, featuring the story of a famous cricket player who had had to stop playing because of panic attacks but who then recovered. The cricketer was played by a soft toy belonging to the client. The techniques the cricketer used to recover were the MAPP techniques that the client had found helpful.
- A PowerPoint presentation featuring different images of useful strategies learned during MAPP.

Step 3: Discuss the Client's Answers to the Core Guide Questions and Plan the Video

The client and therapist(s) begin this step by discussing the client's answers to the core guide questions. This part of the session may also focus on expanding any answers (if needed) before the filming of the blueprint begins. Ideally, the client will have made some notes on the guide questions. The client and therapist(s) can then decide how the video will be structured, who will be in the video, what props will be needed (if any), and so on. For example, the client may want to hold up examples of postcards that he or she has noted strategies on, or representations of visual metaphors.

Step 4: Produce the Video Blueprint

The actual production of the video blueprint is rather straightforward, once the preparation has been completed as described above. We recommend a "test run" to check that the video's quality is good, that the sound is audible, and that the light is adequate. A video typically starts with a brief introduction from either a therapist or the client, stating the date and time when the video is being made, and the purpose of the video.

At the end of the video-making process, we suggest reviewing the first couple of minutes together. Clients are often nervous about how they will appear or sound on video; ideally, seeing the video will allay their fears.

Step 5: Review and Discuss the Blueprint Together in Session

Watching the video together in the next session gives all parties a chance to reflect on the content of the video and the learning that has taken place over the course of the intervention.

Often clients will remark that they did not realize how much they had learned, or that the blueprint procedure helped them to remember important strategies that they would have forgotten otherwise. Following the review of the video, the client is given a copy of the video to take home (unless it is already on the client's phone). It is worth thinking with the client about where to store this video and when to watch it. We encourage clients to look at their videos on a regular basis—perhaps once a month in the first few months after therapy—in order to further consolidate strategies.

Table 12.1 contains a summary of the tasks to be completed in the consolidation sessions, as well as how they are introduced at the end of the active treatment phase of MAPP.

CASE EXAMPLE: JACK

Jack had a current diagnosis of BD Type I and social anxiety disorder/social phobia, as well as a history of PTSD and alcohol use disorder. In the MAPP intervention sessions, he had worked hard to rescript an image that caused him high anxiety. The original image was related to his strained relationship with his extended family, and was associated with feelings of detachment, coldness, rigidity, and indifference. The rescripted "antidote" image he had created to counter this original image was associated with feelings of connectedness, warmth, creativity, and intimacy that he had experienced with some childhood friends.

When the idea of making a video blueprint was raised, Jack was initially reluctant to be videoed. However, he understood the rationale for creating the blueprint and could see the potential value in doing it. He requested that the two cotherapists be included in the video, and that it take the form of a fluid conversation between him and the therapists. Jack

TABLE 12.1. What to Cover in Preparation for and during the Consolidation Sessions

Session	Steps required
At end of final treatment session (treatment session 4)	• Introduce rationale for consolidation sessions. • Discuss procedure. • Give client list of core guide questions to begin thinking through/ making notes on at home in preparation for first consolidation session. • Encourage client to be creative; there is no one way to do a video blueprint.
Consolidation session 1	• Recap procedure for session. • Discuss core guide questions, elicit reflections on questions from client, review any notes client has made, and plan further information to include. • Make video blueprint. • Review first 1–2 minutes of blueprint together. • Elicit client feedback on procedure.
Consolidation session 2	• Obtain client feedback on previous session. • Watch video blueprint in full together in session. • Give client a copy of the blueprint to take home.

used his prepared answers to the core guide questions very well during the making of the blueprint, and he reported afterward that he forgot that he was being videoed at times.

Prior to watching the video with the therapists during consolidation session 2, Jack was understandably anxious. However, on watching the video, he commented that he looked far less nervous than he had expected to.

At one point in the session, the video was paused, and a still image of the two therapists and Jack in conversation was left on the screen. At this moment, Jack spontaneously commented that this image represented many of the same qualities as the rescripted image we had worked to create in therapy: human warmth and connectedness; creative solutions generated by three people working together in collaboration; and a sense of trust and intimacy. As such, this "still" from the video blueprint became another image to remind him of the sessions and the strategies he had learned, which he could bring to mind as and when he needed to.

Hints and Tips for Addressing Clients' Anxiety about Creating Videos

It is highly likely that clients will express anxiety about the idea of being videoed or the prospect of watching themselves or hearing their voices on a video. Therapists can first of all acknowledge that many if not most people feel this way, and that it would be unusual not to feel a little nervous, unless one were a news anchor or something similar.

Most clients will say that they are prepared to give appearing in a video a try, even though it may feel uncomfortable. For those clients who are very anxious about creating a blueprint, therapists can keep these points in mind:

- It may be helpful to reiterate the rationale for creating a blueprint in this way, so that the clients are clear about the potential benefits of the exercise.
- A significant number of people with BD may have some aspects of social anxiety. Therefore, just as in a video feedback session for social anxiety, it can be useful for therapists to ask the clients to state what they think they will see/hear when they watch the video, and how bad or distressing they think this will be on a scale of 0–100%. Once the video has been watched, further ratings can be taken. In our experience, clients typically report a reduction in anxiety once they have watched the video.
- Finally, if a client really does not wish to appear in a video, then this wish should be respected. However, a blueprint should still be made, and the client should be encouraged to collaborate on how best to do this.

CLIENT REFLECTION ON CONSOLIDATION SESSIONS

The following is an observation from a MAPP client who was asked for feedback at the end of treatment. It reflects the usefulness of making a video blueprint.

"In the last sessions, they suggested we make a video describing my MAPP journey. Even though I really dislike being recorded, they persuaded me that, well, making a video would be memorable and would help me cement all I had learned, which was what I wanted too. So I managed to do this, and then they gave it to me on a CD, and

I saved it on my computer. . . . I still have it, and I know exactly where it is on my computer! Yes, it was a stressful process making the video, but by that time I had learned not to be too scared by the challenges of MAPP, and in fact it was really worth it. . . . The memory of the video is like having all of MAPP sealed in my head!"

CONCLUDING COMMENTS

In this chapter, we have covered the final two sessions of the MAPP protocol, which are devoted to consolidation. Using video recording as a novel way of making a blueprint for the future, we aim to help clients really remember what they have learned and to have an easy way of revisiting this should difficulties arise. In our experience, it is an immensely enjoyable and fun part of the treatment, and also one that achieves its purpose.

CHAPTER 13

Final Comments

We have started this volume with background information both on BD and on mental imagery. We have highlighted recommendations from guidance documents for innovative psychological treatments for BD. We have then described how we developed such an intervention in MAPP—marrying what we know about the inner worlds of many people with BD, with simple and effective imagery techniques.

In the bulk of the book, we have gone on to describe in detail how to do the MAPP intervention. We have started with our overarching principles: collaboration; curiosity; a "flat" power hierarchy in the therapeutic relationship; scaffolding of therapy; mood monitoring; and, finally, being kind to oneself. Then, chapter by chapter, we have described how to understand an image in detail and then how to go about choosing an imagery intervention technique. Our aim throughout has been to make the section of the manual on assessment and treatment as user-friendly and helpful as possible. As audience members in teaching workshops, we have always found it most helpful when the trainers tell us the exact words they would use to introduce a topic or show us the exact steps they would take. We have tried to do this for you, our readers, so that you might feel confident to go and try out some imagery techniques yourselves.

Although we have described in detail an intervention that was designed for a client group with BD, we also use all of these techniques in our other clinical work—with clients who have depression, social anxiety disorder/social phobia and other anxiety disorders, OCD, substance misuse, psychosis, and PTSD. Thus we hope that the manual will be of use to people working with clients who experience troubling mental images, whatever their diagnosis or diagnoses.

Finally, all members of the MAPP team agree that they learned a great deal during the development of the intervention. Refining the ins and outs of the various techniques was, of course, very useful. However, what we learned from MAPP about how to approach therapy was probably the most useful lesson of all. There is something about working with imagery that requires therapists to be genuinely curious. Indeed, they cannot be otherwise, because they have no idea what the clients are going to see in their minds, or how they might choose to change this. Therapists also have to be genuinely collaborative, again, because they do not have the answers themselves; the answers lie in the imaginations of their clients. Once we were divested of the need "to know" and to take the lead, we MAPP therapists often found a creativity and playfulness that we did not know we had—which was marvelous, both for us as therapists and for our clients. Yet another thing about working with imagery is that this type of therapy can often achieve profound, emotionally affecting changes in very few sessions. We are excited to anticipate how imagery interventions will be developed and evaluated in the next few years. We encourage you all to have a go at using these interventions. After all, they make you collaborative, curious, and creative, *and* they can precipitate rapid and enduring change. What's not to like?

Good luck.

Afterword

"Since Eve ate apples, much depends on dinner." So said Lord Byron. This book, instead, depended on lunch. About 10 years ago, Emily Holmes, John Geddes, and I regularly met for a sandwich, and sometimes we were joined by Francesc Colom while he was a visiting fellow in Oxford. John and I are psychiatrists with a particular interest in bipolar disorder (BD), and we ran a specialist clinic that served patients with BD. Like Francesc, Emily is a clinical psychologist. Our lunches were serious fun. What we discussed was how psychotherapy could help patients with BD.

John and I were quite uncertain how to advise our patients to seek psychological help. Our main modality of treatment was medication, and picking through the menu of reasonable drug choices to find what suited individual patients was in itself time-consuming, so our own approach to psychological treatment was unambitious: somewhere between interpersonal psychotherapy and simple support (being there).

We were struck that conventionally delivered cognitive-behavioral therapy (CBT), while relatively available locally, was not terribly helpful in BD. Our negative view of conventional CBT was reinforced by a large study led by Jan Scott (Scott et al., 2006), which had been recently published. What our patients said was that the therapists were very nice, but they didn't find that the approach suited them. For example, they didn't feel that they had conscious negative biases, as their therapists clearly expected them to have. Of course, CBT had been developed for patients with unipolar depression, and many practitioners did not accept patients with BD for this reason; however, some did, and some patients had originally presented with depression and not been diagnosed as having BD until after they had received CBT.

Francesc had performed a major study of psychoeducation with Eduard Vieta in Barcelona (Colom et al., 2003). They had demonstrated that a group didactic approach to improving patients' understanding of BD seemed to be significantly better than a supportive nondirective group therapy. Emily brought entirely new ideas about mental imagery to our conversation. They came from her work on trauma-related anxiety and her understanding of cognitive neuroscience. Anxiety was very common in patients with BD—so common that I tended to see it as a core symptom rather than a comorbidity. The work of Jules Angst supported that perspective (Angst et al., 2010). Moreover, severe anxiety seemed to be associated with worse outcomes (Simon et al., 2004). Somehow there had to be a connection among these factors.

The possible (missing) link between imagery and BD occurred to us as a hypothesis worth investigating. It turned out that patients with BD are indeed prone to negative imagery, and Emily and colleagues applied this perspective to developing the treatment approach that ultimately became MAPP. In short, they have shown that by making use of imagery in treatment, CBT practitioners can help patients with BD to manage their anxiety and other symptoms.

The role of CBT in BD remains controversial. There is still a dearth of good evidence, and sometimes there is a willingness to overplay what evidence there is (Jauhar et al., 2016). The responsible consensus has been cautious in recognizing only psychoeducation as the foundation of psychological support in BD (Goodwin et al., 2016). However, the MAPP treatment Emily and her colleagues have developed has shown real promise in patients with BD. Furthermore, it provides a guide to address imagery across diagnoses. It is practical and pragmatic, and I am excited to see it disseminated more widely in this manual.

GUY GOODWIN, FMedSci
Department of Psychiatry
University of Oxford

Appendices

MAPP Information Sheet/Imagery Assessment Guide for Clinicians

What Is Mental Imagery?

Clients report thinking in words and/or images. In assessments, clinicians typically ask about words ("thoughts"; e.g., "Do you have thoughts of harming yourself?"), but don't always ask about images.

A definition of mental imagery from cognitive neuroscience is this: "Mental imagery occurs when perceptual information is accessed from memory, giving rise to the experience of 'seeing with the mind's eye,' 'hearing with the mind's ear,' and so on. By contrast, perception occurs when information is directly registered from the senses."[1]

In clinical reality, what we mean by "mental imagery" is thinking in the forms of mental pictures and images—for example, having a vivid picture in mind of harming oneself, or an intrusive visual memory of a traumatic event.

The following words or phrases used by clients can alert clinicians to mental imagery: "pictures," "flashes," "pop-ins," "like a photo," "I can see myself . . ."

Why Is It Important to Ask about Clients' Mental Imagery?[2]

- Mental imagery has a more powerful impact on emotion than verbal cognition does.
- It also has impacts on learning and behavior.
- It has perceptual equivalence with real experience.
- It is more memorable than words.

Mental Imagery and Psychological Disorders

Mental imagery occurs across a wide range of psychological disorders and is implicated in the etiology and maintenance of symptoms.[3] It is found in the following: bipolar disorder (BD), posttraumatic stress disorder (PTSD), social anxiety disorder/social phobia, agoraphobia, obsessive–compulsive disorder (OCD), depression, psychosis, body dysmorphic disorder (BDD), and substance misuse cravings.

Mental Imagery and Suicide

At times of suicidal ideation/crisis, mental imagery about suicide has been found to be more prominent and compelling (i.e., associated with a wish to act) than verbal thoughts of suicide,[4] particularly in BD (which has the highest suicide rate of all psychiatric disorders). Therefore, mental imagery of suicide may be an important marker of suicide risk/adverse outcome.

(continued)

Why Might Clients Not Spontaneously Tell Therapists about Mental Imagery?

Clients do not tend spontaneously to report mental imagery. Many clients do not notice that they are experiencing mental images until therapists ask about them. Alternatively, clients may be embarrassed, ashamed, disturbed, or disgusted by their imagery; may be unfamiliar with talking about images or memories; or perhaps believe that the imagery is a sign that they are going mad. *Therefore, it is important to assess imagery in addition to verbal cognitions.*

A Brief Guide to Assessing Imagery in Clients

Just as clients vary in their ability to identify verbal thoughts, they also vary in their ability to identify images.

1. *We would therefore recommend defining mental imagery in simple terms for each client.* A very simple explanation might be this: "When you think about that [e.g., committing suicide/memory of trauma], do you ever 'see it in your mind's eye' or see a vivid picture of it?" A more careful explanation might be something like this:

> "When we think, we can do so in two ways: words or 'mental images.' When we think in verbal thoughts, we think in language of the sort we would use when we speak. For instance, a verbal thought about this appointment might be 'This therapist is asking me so many questions!', which would run through your mind as words.
>
> "When we think in mental images, we imagine pictures in the mind's eye. A mental image about this appointment might be picturing in your mind's eye what the room looks like with us sitting in it. Although mental images often take the form of pictures, they can actually include any of the five senses. For example, you could 'hear' the sound of us talking in your imagination. We can also have image memories that come back as smells or sensations. Images can be very clear and vivid, or unclear and fleeting. 'Mental imagery' refers to all these different types of imagining."

2. *Clients may find their mental imagery shaming or disturbing, or may interpret it as a sign of madness.* Therapists should therefore normalize the presence of imagery before inquiring about imagery in detail—for instance, by saying something like this:

> "Many people experience vivid mental images. These can be positive (for example, a memory of a happy event such as a wedding) or negative (such as having nasty images pop into your mind unbidden). We know that up to 90% of the population will experience disturbing images from time to time. Mental imagery can become more prominent at times of emotional stress."

3. *The following questions can be useful for assessing specific imagery in your clients, since they can help focus the clients by first grounding them in a specific time period and context:*

> "When you are feeling depressed/anxious/high, is there a common or repeated image that comes to mind?"

(continued)

"When was the last time you were tearful/jittery/high? Where were you? Did any images come to mind at this time?"

"Does your mental imagery change, depending on how you are feeling? For example, do you notice that you experience different types of mental imagery when you are depressed, compared to when you are anxious [high, etc.]?"

"Which image do you feel is most significant for you? How frequently do you experience this image?"

"If you bring this image to mind now, how does it make you feel?"

"Does the imagery have any meanings associated with it—for example, how you think about yourself or others? How much do you believe the image?"

"Does the imagery make you want to do anything particular in response to it? How compelling is the imagery?"

[1]Kosslyn, Ganis, and Thompson (2001).
[2]Holmes and Mathews (2005).
[3]Hackmann and Holmes (2004).
[4]Holmes et al. (2007); Crane, Shah, Barnhofer, and Holmes (2012); Hales et al. (2011).

Agendas for Each of the 10 Sessions
of the MAPP Protocol

These agendas can be used to guide what to do in each session and can be placed in view between a therapist and client. When a task is complete, the therapist can check off the box in the right-hand column.

AGENDA: Assessment ("Mapping") Session 1

• Turn on recording equipment (if being used).	
• Set agenda.	
• Introduce MAPP model.	
• Describe aim and purpose of mapping sessions.	
• Main agenda items to cover:	
○ Confirm reason for referral.	
○ Review current mood (refer to scores for QIDS, ASRM, and BAI, which ideally have been submitted online).	
○ Ascertain reported client priorities (cross-check with referral letter).	
○ Review medication issues.	
○ Begin to map imagery/comorbidities influencing mood stability.	
○ Begin to note current positive coping strategies.	
• Check that future mapping sessions are scheduled.	

AGENDA: Assessment ("Mapping") Session 2

• Turn on recording equipment (if being used).	
• Set agenda.	
• Review mood (as above).	
• Review information covered in assessment session 1.	
• Main agenda items to cover:	
o Begin life chart—episodes of anxiety, depression, and (hypo)mania mapped above line; life events below.	
o Assess client's ability to identify prodromes of (hypo)mania and depression.	
o Further investigate imagery/comorbidities influencing mood stability.	
o Begin microformulation of imagery, if possible.	
o Add information to other sections in MAPP Assessment ("Mapping") Document (Appendix 3), if any emerges.	
• If appropriate, therapist(s) to select appropriate specific questionnaires for client to fill in, based on information gained (e.g., to assess social anxiety).	
• Assign homework: Client to continue working on life chart, if he or she wishes and this is appropriate.	
• Photocopy life chart for client to take home and work on if he or she wishes.	

AGENDA: Assessment ("Mapping") Session 3

• Turn on recording equipment (if being used).	
• Set agenda.	
• Review mood (briefly).	
• Review specific measures (if applicable).	
• Review homework of completing life chart (if assigned); add further information.	
• Review draft mapping report.	
• Main agenda items to cover:	
○ Client and therapist to jointly amend mapping report.	
○ Refine microformulations of imagery, with aim of identifying concrete intervention targets.	
○ Flesh out other sections of mapping report, if necessary/helpful. (The mapping report is viewed as a document that provides a useful summary of information for the client and other professionals who may be involved in their care. Any further information that the client or therapist perceives as useful should therefore be included.)	

AGENDA: Assessment ("Mapping") Session 4

• Turn on recording equipment (if being used).	
• Set agenda.	
• Review mood (briefly).	
• Review specific measures (if applicable).	
• Review revised mapping report.	
• Main agenda items to cover.	
o Agree on MAPP treatment module target.	
o Seek client feedback on his or her experience of the mapping sessions: What was useful/not useful?	
o Explain MAPP treatment procedure.	
• Confirm dates for MAPP treatment module.	

AGENDA: Treatment Session 1

• Turn on recording equipment (if being used).	
• Set agenda.	
• Review mood (briefly), and complete measures if not done online.	
• Confirm imagery target.	
• Expand imagery microformulation if necessary.	
• Decide which active treatment technique is needed of the following:	
○ Rescripting imagery.	
○ Promoting positive imagery.	
○ Imagery-competing tasks.	
○ Metacognitive techniques to reduce power of the image.	
• Explain rationale for active technique, and begin.	
• Assign homework (if appropriate).	

AGENDA: Treatment Session 2

• Turn on recording equipment (if being used).	
• Set agenda.	
• Review mood (briefly), and complete measures if not done online.	
• Cover specific items, depending on imagery target:	
• Assign homework (if appropriate).	

AGENDA: Treatment Session 3

• Turn on recording equipment (if being used).	
• Set agenda.	
• Review mood (briefly), and complete measures if not done online.	
• Cover specific items, depending on imagery target:	
• Assign homework (if appropriate).	

AGENDA: Treatment Session 4

• Turn on recording equipment (if being used).	
• Set agenda.	
• Review mood (briefly), and complete measures if not done online.	
• Cover specific items, depending on imagery target:	
• Complete imagery work.	
• Introduce rationale for consolidation sessions.	
• Discuss video blueprint procedure.	
• Give client the list of core guide questions to begin thinking through/making notes on at home in preparation for first consolidation session.	
• Encourage client to be creative (no one way to do video blueprint).	

AGENDA: Consolidation Session 1

• Turn on recording equipment (if being used).	
• Set agenda.	
• Review mood (briefly), and complete measures if not done online.	
• Discuss draft end-of-treatment report.	
• Recap procedure for session.	
• Discuss core guide questions, elicit reflections on questions from client, review any notes made, and plan further information to include.	
• Make video blueprint.	
• Review first 1–2 minutes of blueprint together.	
• Elicit client feedback on procedure, and give positive reinforcement for completing it.	

AGENDA: Consolidation Session 2

• Turn on recording equipment (if being used).	
• Set agenda.	
• Review mood (briefly), and complete measures if not done online.	
• Obtain client feedback on previous session.	
• Watch video blueprint in full together in session.	
• Give client a copy of the blueprint to take home.	
• Reflect on MAPP sessions as a whole.	

MAPP Assessment ("Mapping") Document

Client's name: _____

Before the client arrives:
- Tidy up environment to reduce overstimulation.
- Have glass of water and tissues ready.
- Review recent contacts.
- Review previous mood data if available.

1. Reason for referral; client's reported priorities:

2. Medication issues:

3. Life chart:

4. Positive coping strategies:

(continued)

5. Ability to identify prodromes of (hypo)mania and depression:

    a. (Hypo)mania:

    b. Depression:

6. Assessment of imagery/comorbidities influencing mood stability:

7. Initial microformulation of imagery (see Appendix 4):

8. Selection of treatment target(s):

9. Any other notes (e.g., liaison with psychiatrist over mapping sessions):

Print out this form and use it to record information during the assessment/"mapping" sessions.

Microformulation Template

This is filled out jointly with the therapist(s) during the assessment phase of the intervention and is used to help identify which intervention strategies to use.

(continued)

Microformulation Template *(page 2 of 2)*

Original source

[ ]

⬇

Trigger(s)

[ ]

⬇

Image description

[ ]

What is it of?

Maintaining factors for persistence of image

[ ]

How do you behave/what do you have to do/how do you cope because of this implication?

Emotion(s) in image

(Congruence)

⬌

How do you feel?

Appraisal(s) in image

What are you thinking?

Power of the image: Why is it not dismissed?

[ ]

For example:
What do you have to do because of it behaviorally/ cognitively?
What does it mean about you that you have this image?
Do you believe it? Is it true/real/prophetic?

Bring to mind recent example

Chart for Recording Emotions and Appraisals within a Troublesome Image

For the target image, fill in the emotion(s) that you feel while you hold it in mind. Then establish what you are thinking/what is running through your mind that is making you feel that emotion. Ensure that you establish this information for *all* of the emotions that you feel when you hold the image in mind.

Image	Emotions: How do you feel?	Appraisals: When you feel X, what is running through your mind? What are you thinking that is making you feel X?

Chart for Recording the Meaning of a Troublesome Image

For the target image, transfer information (gained during the microformulation stage) into this chart about the emotions and appraisals in the image. Then rate the intensity of the emotions (0–100%). Finally, think about the meaning of the image—the combination of how it makes you feel, what you are thinking, and the power of the image. Together, these things form the meaning of the image and will explain why you react to it in the way that you do. Rate how much you believe this meaning (0–100%) *while the image is in your mind*, not how much you believe it later.

Image	Emotions: How do you feel?	Appraisals: When you feel X, what is running through your mind? What are you thinking that is making you feel X? Rate intensity of emotions: 0% (no emotion)–100% (most intense emotions ever experienced).	Meanings: What is it that you believe or know or feel that explains the way you react to the image? Rate how much you believe each meaning: 0% (do not believe at all)–100% (completely believe).

Chart for Constructing an Antidote for a Troublesome Image

For the target image, transfer information into this chart about the emotions and meanings in the image. Then think about what emotions would be the opposites/the "antidotes" to the "toxic" emotions. Next, think about what meanings would generate those antidote emotions. Remember, you may need to address *all* aspects of a toxic meaning with an antidote: toxic emotions, toxic appraisals, and the perceived power of the image. Rate how much you believe the antidote meanings (0–100%). Finally, generate an antidote image to try out—one that encapsulates the antidote meanings and generates the antidote emotions.

Image	Emotions: How do you feel?	Meanings: What is it that you believe or know or feel that explains the way you react to the image? Rate how much you believe each meaning: 0% (do not believe at all)–100% (completely believe).	Antidote Emotions: What would be the antidote to that feeling?	Antidote Meanings: What would you have to know or believe to experience this antidote feeling? (Note: This needs to counter *all* of the meaning, including the power of the image.) Rate how much you believe each antidote meaning: 0% (do not believe at all)–100% (completely believe).	Antidote Image: What image springs to mind/can we construct that incorporates the antidote meaning and will make you feel the antidote emotions?

Chart for Monitoring Progress in Practicing an Antidote Image

Write a brief description of the antidote image, and then rate (on a scale of 0–100%) the intensity of the antidote emotions generated as you practice the antidote image. Also rate how vivid the image is, on the same scale.

Antidote Image	Antidote Emotions and Vividness Rate intensity of antidote emotions and vividness of image: 0–100%.		
	Practice 1	Practice 2	Practice 3

Chart for Monitoring Progress in Practicing a Positive Image

Write a brief description of the positive image, and then rate (on a scale of 0–100%) the intensity of the target emotions generated as you practice the image. Also rate how vivid the image is, on the same scale.

Positive Image	Target Positive Emotions and Vividness of Image Rate intensity of target emotions and vividness of image: 0–100%.						
	Practice 1	Practice 2	Practice 3	Practice 4	Practice 5	Practice 6	Practice 7

Chart for Monitoring Progress in Using Imagery-Competing Tasks

Note down when you used the task and which task you used. Rate the vividness and distress of the troublesome image(s) *before the competing task* (on a scale of 0–100%, where 0% = not at all vivid/no distress and 100% = extremely vivid/distressing). Then rerate how vivid/distressing the image is, on the same scale, after the competing task.

Day and time of practice	Visuospatial task used	Vividness of image(s) before (0–100%)	Distress of image(s) before (0–100%)	Vividness of image(s) after (0–100%)	Distress of image(s) after (0–100%)

References

Alloy, L. B., Bender, R. E., Whitehouse, W. G., Wagner, C. A., Liu, R. T., Grant, D. A., et al. (2012). High behavioral approach system (BAS) sensitivity, reward responsiveness, and goal-striving predict first onset of bipolar spectrum disorders: A prospective behavioral high-risk design. *Journal of Abnormal Psychology, 121*(2), 339–351.

Altman, E. G., Hedeker, D., Peterson, J. L., & Davis, J. M. (1997). The Altman Self-Rating Mania Scale. *Biological Psychiatry, 42*(10), 948–955.

American Psychiatric Association. (2002). Practice guideline for the treatment of patients with bipolar disorder (rev.). *American Journal of Psychiatry, 159*(4, Suppl.), 1–50.

American Psychiatric Association. (2013). *Diagnostic and statistical manual of mental disorders* (5th ed.). Arlington, VA: Author.

Angst, J., Cui, L., Swendsen, J., Rothen, S., Cravchik, A., Kessler, R. C., et al. (2010). Major depressive disorder with subthreshold bipolarity in the National Comorbidity Survey Replication. *American Journal of Psychiatry, 167*, 1194–1201.

Arntz, A., & Jacob, G. A. (2013). *Schema therapy in practice: An introductory guide to the schema mode approach.* Oxford, UK: Wiley-Blackwell.

Arntz, A., Sofi, D., & van Breukelen, G. (2013). Imagery rescripting as a treatment for complicated PTSD in refugees: A multiple baseline case series study. *Behaviour Research and Therapy, 51*(6), 274–283.

Arntz, A., Tiesema, M., & Kindt, M. (2007). Treatment of PTSD: A comparison of imaginal exposure with and without imagery rescripting. *Journal of Behavior Therapy and Experimental Psychiatry, 38*(4), 345–370.

Aronson, J., Fried, C. B., & Good, C. (2002). Reducing the effects of stereotype threat on African American college students by shaping theories of intelligence. *Journal of Experimental Social Psychology, 38*, 113–125.

Baldessarini, R. J., Faedda, G. L., Offidani, E., Vazquez, G. H., Marangoni, C., Serra, G., et al. (2013). Antidepressant-associated mood-switching and transition from unipolar major depression to bipolar disorder: A review. *Journal of Affective Disorders, 148*(1), 129–135.

Beck, A. T. (1970). Cognitive therapy: Nature and relation to behavior therapy. *Behavior Therapy, 1*(2), 184–200.

Beck, A. T., Brown, G., Epstein, N., & Steer, R. A. (1988). An inventory for measuring clinical anxiety: Psychometric properties. *Journal of Consulting and Clinical Psychology, 56*(6), 893–897.

Beck, A. T., & Emery, G., with Greenberg, R. L. (1985). *Anxiety disorders and phobias: A cognitive perspective.* New York: Basic Books.

Beck, J. S. (2005). *Cognitive therapy for challenging problems: What to do when the basics don't work.* New York: Guilford Press.

Birmaher, B., Gill, M. K., Axelson, D. A., Goldstein, B. I., Goldstein, T. R., Yu, H., et al. (2014). Longitudinal trajectories and associated baseline predictors in youths with bipolar spectrum disorders. *American Journal of Psychiatry, 171*(9), 990–999.

Blackwell, S. E., Browning, M., Mathews, A., Pictet, A., Welch, J., Davies, J., et al. (2015).

Positive imagery-based cognitive bias modification as a web-based treatment for depressed adults: A randomized controlled trial. *Clinical Psychological Science, 3*(1), 91–111.

Blackwell, S. E., & Holmes, E. A. (2010). Modifying interpretation and imagination in clinical depression: A single case series using cognitive bias modification. *Applied Cognitive Psychology, 24*(3), 338–350.

Bopp, J. M., Miklowitz, D. J., Goodwin, G. M., Rendell, J. M., & Geddes, J. R. (2010). The longitudinal course of bipolar disorder as revealed through weekly text messaging: A feasibility study. *Bipolar Disorders, 12*(3), 327–334.

Brewin, C. R., Watson, M., McCarthy, S., Hyman, P., & Dayson, D. (1998). Intrusive memories and depression in cancer patients. *Behaviour Research and Therapy, 36*(12), 1131–1142.

Carstenson, B. (1955). The auxiliary chair technique: A case study. *Group Psychotherapy, 8,* 50–56.

Cassidy, F., Ahearn, E. P., & Carroll, B. J. (2001). Substance abuse in bipolar disorder. *Bipolar Disorders, 3*(4), 181–188.

Chatterton, M. L., Stockings, E., Berk, M., Barendregt, J. J., Carter, R., & Mihalopoulos, C. (2017). Psychosocial therapies for the adjunctive treatment of bipolar disorder in adults: Network meta-analysis. *British Journal of Psychiatry, 210*(5), 333–341.

Colom, F., & Lam, D. (2005). Psychoeducation: Improving outcomes in bipolar disorder. *European Psychiatry, 20*(5–6), 359–364.

Colom, F., & Vieta, E. (2006). *Psychoeducation manual for bipolar disorder.* Cambridge, UK: Cambridge University Press.

Colom, F., Vieta, E., Martinez-Aran, A., Reinares, M., Goikolea, J. M., Benabarre, A., et al. (2003). A randomized trial on the efficacy of group psychoeducation in the prophylaxis of recurrences in bipolar patients whose disease is in remission. *Archives of General Psychiatry, 60,* 402–407.

Colom, F., Vieta, E., Sánchez-Moreno, J., Palomino-Otiniano, R., Reinares, M., Goikolea, J. M., et al. (2009). Group psychoeducation for stabilised bipolar disorders: 5-year outcome of a randomised clinical trial. *British Journal of Psychiatry, 194*(3), 260–265.

Crane, C., Shah, D., Barnhofer, T., & Holmes, E. A. (2012). Suicidal imagery in a previously depressed community sample. *Clinical Psychology and Psychotherapy, 19*(1), 57–69.

Crowe, M., Beaglehole, B., & Inder, M. (2016). Social rhythm interventions for bipolar disorder: A systematic review and rationale for practice. *Journal of Psychiatric and Mental Health Nursing, 23*(1), 3–11.

Cumming, J., & Ramsey, R. (2008). Sport imagery interventions. In S. Mellalieu & S. Hanton (Eds.), *Advances in applied sport psychology: A review* (pp. 5–36). London: Routledge.

de Silva, P. (1986). Obsessional–compulsive imagery. *Behaviour Research and Therapy, 24*(3), 333–350.

Decety, J., & Grèzes, J. (2006). The power of simulation: Imagining one's own and other's behavior. *Brain Research, 1079*(1), 4–14.

Deeprose, C., & Holmes, E. A. (2010). An exploration of prospective imagery: The Impact of Future Events Scale. *Behavioural and Cognitive Psychotherapy, 38*(2), 201–209.

Di Simplicio, M., Renner, F., Blackwell, S. E., Mitchell, H., Stratford, H. J., Watson, P., et al. (2016). An investigation of mental imagery in bipolar disorder: Exploring "the mind's eye." *Bipolar Disorders, 18*(8), 669–683.

Ehlers, A., & Clark, D. M. (2000). A cognitive model of posttraumatic stress disorder. *Behaviour Research and Therapy, 38*(4), 319–345.

Ehlers, A., Clark, D. M., Hackmann, A., McManus, F., Fennell, M., Herbert, C., et al. (2003). A randomized controlled trial of cognitive therapy, a self-help booklet, and repeated assessments as early interventions for posttraumatic stress disorder. *Archives of General Psychiatry, 60*(10), 1024–1032.

Engelhard, I. M., van den Hout, M. A., Janssen, W. C., & van der Beek, J. (2010). Eye movements reduce vividness and emotionality of "flashforwards." *Behaviour Research and Therapy, 48*(5), 442–447.

Fagiolini, A., Frank, E., Rucci, P., Cassano, G. B., Turkin, S., & Kupfer, D. J. (2007). Mood and anxiety spectrum as a means to identify clinically relevant subtypes of bipolar I disorder. *Bipolar Disorders, 9*(5), 462–467.

Foa, E. B., & Rothbaum, B. O. (1998). *Treating the trauma of rape: Cognitive-behavioral therapy for PTSD.* New York: Guilford Press.

Forty, L., Smith, D., Jones, L., Jones, I., Caesar, S., Cooper, C., et al. (2008). Clinical differences between bipolar and unipolar depression. *British Journal of Psychiatry, 192*(5), 388–389.

Fountoulakis, K. N., Grunze, H., Vieta, E.,

Young, A., Yatham, L., Blier, P., et al. (2017). The International College of Neuro-Psychopharmacology (CINP) treatment guidelines for bipolar disorder in adults (CINP-BD-2017), Part 3: The clinical guidelines. *International Journal of Neuropsychopharmacology, 20*(2), 180–195.

Frank, E. (Ed.). (2005). *Treating bipolar disorder: A clinician's guide to interpersonal and social rhythm therapy.* New York: Guilford Press.

Frank, E., Kupfer, D. J., Thase, M. E., Mallinger, A. G., Swartz, H. A., Fagiolini, A. M., et al. (2005). Two-year outcomes for interpersonal and social rhythm therapy in individuals with bipolar I disorder. *Archives of General Psychiatry, 62*(9), 996–1004.

Freeman, M. P., Freeman, S. A., & McElroy, S. L. (2002). The comorbidity of bipolar and axiety disorders: Prevalence, psychobiology, and treatment issues. *Journal of Affective Disorders, 68*(1), 1–12.

Geddes, J. R., & Miklowitz, D. J. (2013). Treatment of bipolar disorder. *Lancet, 381*, 1672–1682.

Gilbert, P. (2009). *The compassionate mind.* London: Constable & Robinson.

Gilbert, P., & Irons, C. (2005). Focused therapies and compassionate mind training for shame and self-attacking. In P. Gilbert (Ed.), *Compassion: Conceptualisations, research and use in psychotherapy* (pp. 263–322). London: Routledge.

Goldberg, J. F., & Garno, J. L. (2005). Development of posttraumatic stress disorder in adult bipolar patients with histories of severe childhood abuse. *Journal of Psychiatric Research, 39*(6), 595–601.

Goldfried, M. R. (1988). Application of rational restructuring to anxiety disorders. *The Counseling Psychologist, 16*, 50–68.

Goodwin, G. M., Haddad, P. M., Ferrier, I. N., Aronson, J. K., Barnes, T., Cipriani, A., et al. (2016). Evidence-based guidelines for treating bipolar disorder: Revised third edition recommendations from the British Association for Psychopharmacology. *Journal of Psychopharmacology, 30*(6), 495–553.

Greitemeyer, T., & Wurz, D. (2006). Mental simulation and the achievement of health goals: The role of goal difficulty. *Imagination, Cognition and Personality, 25*, 239–251.

Grey, N., Young, K., & Holmes, E. A. (2002). Cognitive restructuring within reliving: A treatment for peritraumatic emotional "hotspots" in posttraumatic stress disorder. *Behavioural and Cognitive Psychotherapy, 30*(1), 37–56.

Hackmann, A., Bennett-Levy, J., & Holmes, E. A. (2011). *Oxford guide to imagery in cognitive therapy.* Oxford, UK: Oxford University Press.

Hackmann, A., & Holmes, E. A. (2004). Reflecting on imagery: A clinical perspective and overview of the special issue of *Memory* on mental imagery and memory in psychopathology. *Memory, 12*(4), 389–402.

Hales, S. A., Blackwell, S. E., Di Simplicio, M., Iyadurai, L., Young, K., & Holmes, E. A. (2015). Imagery-based cognitive-behavioral assessment. In G. P. Brown & D. A. Clark (Eds.), *Assessment in cognitive therapy* (pp. 69–93). New York: Guilford Press.

Hales, S. A., Deeprose, C., Goodwin, G. M., & Holmes, E. A. (2011). Cognitions in bipolar disorder versus unipolar depression: Imagining suicide. *Bipolar Disorders, 13*(7–8), 651–661.

Hales, S. A., DiSimplicio, M., Lyadurai, L., Blackwell, S. E., Young, K., Fairburn, C. G., et al. (2018). Imagery-focused cognitive therapy (ImCT) for mood instability and anxiety in a small sample of patients with bipolar disorder: A pilot clinical audit. *Behavioural and Cognitive Psychotherapy, 46*(6), 706–725.

Hawton, K., Sutton, L., Haw, C., Sinclair, J., & Harriss, L. (2005). Suicide and attempted suicide in bipolar disorder: A systematic review of risk factors. *Journal of Clinical Psychiatry, 66*(6), 693–704.

Henry, C., Van den Bulke, D., Bellivier, F., Roy, I., Swendsen, J., M'Baïlara, K., et al. (2008). Affective lability and affect intensity as core dimensions of bipolar disorders during euthymic period. *Psychiatry Research, 159*(1–2), 1–6.

Hirschfeld, R. M., Calabrese, J. R., Frye, M. A., Lavori, P. W., Sachs, G., Thase, M. E., et al. (2007). Defining the clinical course of bipolar disorder: Response, remission, relapse, recurrence, and roughening. *Psychopharmacology Bulletin, 40*(3), 7–14.

Holmes, E. A., Arntz, A., & Smucker, M. R. (2007). Imagery rescripting in cognitive behaviour therapy: Images, treatment techniques and outcomes. *Journal of Behavior Therapy and Experimental Psychiatry, 38*(4), 297–305.

Holmes, E. A., Blackwell, S. E., Burnett Heyes, S., Renner, F., & Raes, F. (2016). Mental imagery in depression: Phenomenology, potential mechanisms, and treatment implications.

Annual Review of Clinical Psychology, 12, 249–280.

Holmes, E. A., Bonsall, M. B., Hales, S. A., Mitchell, H., Renner, F., & Blackwell, S. E., (2016). Applications of time-series analysis to mood fluctuations in bipolar disorder to promote treatment innovation: A case series. *Translational Psychiatry, 6,* e720.

Holmes, E. A., Deeprose, C., Fairburn, C. G., Wallace-Hadrill, S. M. A., Bonsall, M. B., Geddes, J. R., et al. (2011). Mood stability versus mood instability in bipolar disorder: A possible role for emotional mental imagery. *Behaviour Research and Therapy, 49*(10), 707–713.

Holmes, E. A., Geddes, J. R., Colom, F., & Goodwin, G. M. (2008). Mental imagery as an emotional amplifier: Application to bipolar disorder. *Behaviour Research and Therapy, 46*(12), 1251–1258.

Holmes, E. A., Ghaderi, A., Harmer, C., Ramchandani, P. G., Cuijpers, P., Morrison, A. P., et al. (2018). The *Lancet Psychiatry* Commission on Psychological Treatments Research in Tomorrow's Science. *Lancet Psychiatry, 5*(3), 237–286.

Holmes, E. A., James, E. L., Coode-Bate, T., & Deeprose, C. (2009). Can playing the computer game "Tetris" reduce the build-up of flashbacks for trauma?: A proposal from cognitive science. *PLOS ONE, 4*(1), e4153.

Holmes, E. A., Lang, T. J., Moulds, M. L., & Steele, A. M. (2008). Prospective and positive mental imagery deficits in dysphoria. *Behaviour Research and Therapy, 46*(8), 976–981.

Holmes, E. A., & Mathews, A. (2005). Mental imagery and emotion: A special relationship? *Emotion, 5*(4), 489–497.

Holmes, E. A., & Mathews, A. (2010). Mental imagery in emotion and emotional disorders. *Clinical Psychology Review, 30*(3), 349–367.

Holmes, E. A., Mathews, A., Dalgleish, T., & Mackintosh, B. (2006). Positive interpretation training: Effects of mental imagery versus verbal training on positive mood. *Behavior Therapy, 37*(3), 237–247.

Holmes, E. A., Mathews, A., Mackintosh, B., & Dalgleish, T. (2008). The causal effect of mental imagery on emotion assessed using picture-word cues. *Emotion, 8*(3), 395–409.

Hunt, M. G., & Fenton, M. (2007). Imagery rescripting versus *in vivo* exposure in the treatment of snake fear. *Journal of Behavior Therapy and Experimental Psychiatry, 38*(4), 329–344.

Ivins, A., Di Simplicio, M., Close, H., Goodwin, G. M., & Holmes, E. A. (2014). Mental imagery in bipolar affective disorder versus unipolar depression: Investigating cognitions at times of "positive" mood. *Journal of Affective Disorders, 166,* 234–242.

Iyadurai, L., Blackwell, S. B., Meiser-Stedman, R., Watson, P. C., Bonsall, M. B., Geddes, J. R., et al. (2018). Preventing intrusive memories after trauma via a brief intervention involving Tetris computer game play in the emergency department: A proof-of-concept randomized controlled trial. *Molecular Psychiatry, 23*(3), 674–682.

James, E. L., Bonsall, M. B., Hoppitt, L., Tunbridge, E. M., Geddes, J. R., Milton, A. L., et al. (2015). Computer game play reduces intrusive memories of experimental trauma via reconsolidation update mechanisms. *Psychological Science, 26*(8), 1201–1215.

Jauhar, S., McKenna, P. J., & Laws, K. R. (2016). NICE guidance on psychological treatments for bipolar disorder: Searching for the evidence. *Lancet Psychiatry, 3*(4), 386–388.

Ji, J. L., Burnett Heyes, S., MacLeod, C., & Holmes, E. A. (2016). Emotional mental imagery as simulation of reality: Fear and beyond: A tribute to Peter Lang. *Behavior Therapy, 47*(5), 702–719.

Jones, L., & Stuth, G. (1997). The uses of mental imagery in athletics: An overview. *Applied and Preventive Psychology, 6*(2), 101–115.

Jones, S. H., Smith, G., Mulligan, L. D., Lobban, F., Law, H., Dunn, G., et al. (2015). Recovery-focused cognitive–behavioural therapy for recent-onset bipolar disorder: Randomised controlled pilot trial. *British Journal of Psychiatry, 206*(1), 58–66.

Judd, L. L., Akiskal, H. S., Schetteler, P. J., Endicott, J., Maser, J., Solomon, D. A., et al. (2002). The long-term natural history of the weekly symptomatic status of bipolar I disorder. *Archives of General Psychiatry, 59*(6), 530–537.

Jung, K., & Steil, R. (2013). A randomized controlled trial on cognitive restructuring and imagery modification to reduce the feeling of being contaminated in adult survivors of childhood sexual abuse suffering from posttraumatic stress disorder. *Psychotherapy and Psychosomatics, 82*(4), 213–220.

Kavanagh, D. J., Andrade, J., & May, J. (2005). Imaginary relish and exquisite torture: The elaborated intrusion theory of desire. *Psychological Review, 112*(2), 446–467.

Kavanagh, D. J., Freese, S., Andrade, J., & May, J. (2001). Effects of visuospatial tasks on desensitization to emotive memories. *British Journal of Clinical Psychology, 40*(3), 267–280.

Kessing, L. V., Hansen, M. G., & Andersen, P. K. (2004). Course of illness in depressive and bipolar disorders: Naturalistic study, 1994–1999. *British Journal of Psychiatry, 185*, 372–377.

Knowles, R., Tai, S., Jones, S. H., Highfield, J., Morriss, R., & Bentall, R. P. (2007). Stability of self-esteem in bipolar disorder: Comparisons among remitted bipolar patients, remitted unipolar patients and healthy controls. *Bipolar Disorders, 9*(5), 490–495.

Korrelboom, K., de Jong, M., Huijbrechts, I., & Daansen, P. (2009). Competitive Memory Training (COMET) for treating low self-esteem in patients with eating disorders: A randomized clinical trial. *Journal of Consulting and Clinical Psychology, 77*(5), 974–980.

Korrelboom, K., Marissen, M., & van Assendelft, T. (2011). Competitive Memory Training (COMET) for low self-esteem in patients with personality disorders: A randomized effectiveness study. *Behavioural and Cognitive Psychotherapy, 39*(1), 1–19.

Korrelboom, K., Van der Gaag, M., Hendriks, V. M., Huijbrechts, I., & Berretty, E. W. (2008). Treating obsessions with Competitive Memory Training: A pilot study. *Behavior Therapist, 31*(2), 31–36.

Korrelboom, K., van der Weele, K., Gjaltema, M., & Hoogstraten, C. (2009). Competitive Memory Training (COMET) for treating low self-esteem: A pilot study in a routine clinical setting. *Behavior Therapist, 32*, 3–9.

Kosslyn, S. M., Ganis, G., & Thompson, W. L. (2001). Neural foundations of imagery. *Nature Reviews Neuroscience, 2*(9), 635–642.

Koster, E. H. W., Fox, E., & MacLeod, C. (2009). Introduction to the special section on cognitive bias modification in emotional disorders. *Journal of Abnormal Psychology, 118*(1), 1–4.

Kroon, J. S., Wohlfarth, T. D., Dieleman, J., Sutterland, A. L., Storosum, J. G., Denys, D., et al. (2013). Incidence rates and risk factors of bipolar disorder in the general population: A population-based cohort study. *Bipolar Disorders, 15*(3), 306–313.

Kupka, R. W., Altshuler, L. L., Nolen, W. A., Suppes, T., Luckenbaugh, D. A., Leverich, G. S., et al. (2007). Three times more days depressed than manic or hypomanic in both bipolar I and bipolar II disorder. *Bipolar Disorders, 9*(5), 531–535.

Lam, D. H., Hayward, P., Watkins, E. R., Wright, K., & Sham, P. (2005). Relapse prevention in patients with bipolar disorder: Cognitive therapy outcome after 2 years. *American Journal of Psychiatry, 162*(2), 324–329.

Lam, D. H., Jones, S. H., & Hayward, P. (2010). *Cognitive therapy for bipolar disorder: A therapist's guide to concepts, methods and practice* (2nd ed.). Chichester, UK: Wiley.

Lang, P. J. (1977). Imagery in therapy: An information processing analysis of fear. *Behavior Therapy, 8*(5), 862–886.

Layden, M. A., Newman, C. F., Freeman, A., & Byers Morse, S. (1993). *Cognitive therapy of borderline personality disorder.* Boston: Allyn & Bacon.

Lee, D. A. (2005). The perfect nurturer: A model to develop a compassionate mind within the context of cognitive therapy. In P. Gilbert (Ed.), *Compassion: Conceptualisations, research and use in psychotherapy* (pp. 326–351). London: Routledge.

Lee, D. A., & James, S. (2012). *The compassionate mind approach to recovering from trauma.* London: Robinson.

Lewis, P. A., & Critchley, H. D. (2003). Mood dependent memory. *Trends in Cognitive Sciences, 7*(10), 431–433.

Lilley, S. A., Andrade, J., Turpin, G., Sabin-Farrell, R., & Holmes, E. A. (2009). Visuospatial working memory interference with recollections of trauma. *British Journal of Clinical Psychology, 48*(3), 309–321.

MacLeod, C., Coates, C., & Hetherton, J. (2008). Increasing well-being through teaching and goal-setting and planning skills: Results of a brief intervention. *Journal of Happiness Studies, 9*, 185–196.

MacLeod, C., Koster, E. H. W., & Fox, E. (2009). Whither cognitive bias modification research?: Commentary on the special section articles. *Journal of Abnormal Psychology, 118*(1), 89–99.

Mahlberg, R., Kienast, T., Bschor, T., & Adli, M.

(2008). Evaluation of time memory in acutely depressed patients, manic patients, and healthy controls using a time reproduction task. *European Psychiatry, 23*(6), 430–433.

Malhi, G. S., Ivanovski, B., Hadzi-Pavlovic, D., Mitchell, P. B., Vieta, E., & Sachdev, P. (2007). Neuropsychological deficits and functional impairment in bipolar depression, hypomania and euthymia. *Bipolar Disorders, 9*(1–2), 114–125.

Malik, A., Goodwin, G. M., Hoppitt, L., & Holmes, E. A. (2014). Hypomanic experience in young adults confers vulnerability to intrusive imagery after experimental trauma: Relevance for bipolar disorder. *Clinical Psychological Science, 2*(6), 675–684.

Martínez-Arán, A., Vieta, E., Colom, F., Torrent, C., Sánchez-Moreno, J., Reinares, M., et al. (2004). Cognitive impairment in euthymic bipolar patients: Implications for clinical and functional outcome. *Bipolar Disorders, 6*(3), 224–232.

Merikangas, K. R., Akiskal, H. S., Angst, J., Greenberg, P. E., Hirschfeld, R. M., Petukhova, M., et al. (2007). Lifetime and 12-month prevalence of bipolar spectrum disorder in the National Comorbity Survey Replication. *Archives of General Psychiatry, 64*(5), 543–552.

Merikangas, K. R., Jin, R., He, J. P., Kessler, R. C., Lee, S., Sampson, N. A., et al. (2011). Prevalence and correlates of bipolar spectrum disorder in the World Mental Health Survey initiative. *Archives of General Psychiatry, 68*(3), 241–251.

Miklowitz, D. J., Cipriani, A., & Goodwin, G. M. (2017). Network meta-analysis: Drawing conclusions regarding trials of psychosocial interventions for bipolar disorder. *British Journal of Psychiatry, 211*(6), 334–336.

Miklowitz, D. J., Goodwin, G. M., Bauer, M. S., & Geddes, J. R. (2008). Common and specific elements of psychosocial treatments for bipolar disorder: A survey of clinicians participating in randomized trials. *Journal of Psychiatric Practice, 14*, 77–85.

Miklowitz, D. J., O'Brien, M. P., Schlosser, D. A., Addington, J., Candan, K. A., Marshall, C., et al. (2014). Family-focused treatment for adolescents and young adults at high risk for psychosis: Results of a randomized trial. *Journal of the American Academy of Child and Adolescent Psychiatry, 53*(8), 848–858.

Miklowitz, D. J., Price, J., Holmes, E. A., Rendell, J., Bell, S., Budge, K., et al. (2012). Facilitated integrated mood management for adults with bipolar disorder. *Bipolar Disorders, 14*(2), 185–197.

Morina, N., Lancee, J., & Arntz, A. (2017). Imagery rescripting as a clinical intervention for aversive memories: A meta-analysis. *Journal of Behavior Therapy and Experimental Psychiatry, 55*, 6–15.

Morrison, A. P., Beck, A. T., Glentworth, D., Dunn, H., Reid, G. S., Larkin, W., et al. (2002). Imagery and psychotic symptoms: A preliminary investigation. *Behaviour Research and Therapy, 40*(9), 1053–1062.

Müller-Oerlinghausen, B., Berghöfer, A., & Bauer, M. (2002). Bipolar disorder. *Lancet, 359*(9302), 241–247.

Muse, K., McManus, F., Hackmann, A., & Williams, M. (2010). Intrusive imagery in severe health anxiety: Prevalence, nature and links with memories and maintenance cycles. *Behaviour Research and Therapy, 48*(8), 792–798.

Nandi, A., Beard, J. R., & Galea, S. (2009). Epidemiologic heterogeneity of common mood and anxiety disorders over the lifecourse in the general population: A systematic review. *BMC Psychiatry, 9*(31), 1–11.

National Institute for Health and Care Excellence (NICE). (2014). Bipolar disorder: Assessment and management. Clinical guideline (CG125). Retrieved from *www.nice.org.uk/guidance/cg185/resources/bipolar-disorder-assessment-and-management-35109814379461.*

Ng, R. M. K., Burnett Heyes, S., McManus, F., Kennerley, H., & Holmes, E. A. (2016). Bipolar risk and mental imagery susceptibility in a representative sample of Chinese adults residing in the coummunity. *International Journal of Social Psychiatry, 62*(1), 94–102.

Ng, R. M. K., Di Simplicio, M., McManus, F., Kennerley, H., & Holmes, E. A. (2016). "Flashforwards" and suicidal ideation: A prospective investigation of mental imagery, entrapment and defeat in a cohort from the Hong Kong Mental Morbidity Survey. *Psychiatry Research, 246*, 453–460.

O'Donnell, C., Di Simplicio, M., Brown, R., Holmes, E. A., & Burnett Heyes, S. (2018). The role of mental imagery in mood amplification: An investigation across subclinical features of bipolar disorders. *Cortex, 105*, 104–117.

Osman, S., Cooper, M., Hackmann, A., & Veale,

D. (2004). Spontaneously occuring images and early memories in people with body dysmorphic disorder. *Memory, 12*(4), 428–436.

Otto, M. W., Simon, N. M., Wisniewski, S. R., Miklowitz, D. J., Kogan, J. N., Reilly-Harrington, N. A., et al. (2006). Prospective 12-month course of bipolar disorder in out-patients with and without comorbid anxiety disorders. *British Journal of Psychiatry, 189*(1), 20–25.

Pacchiarotti, I., Bond, D. J., Baldessarini, R. J., Nolen, W. A., Grunze, H., Licht, R. W., et al. (2013). The International Society for Bipolar Disorders (ISBD) task force report on antidepressant use in bipolar disorders. *American Journal of Psychiatry, 170*(11), 1249–1262.

Pavlova, B., Perlis, R. H., Alda, M., & Uher, R. (2015). Lifetime prevalence of anxiety disorders in people with bipolar disorder: A systematic review and meta-analysis. *Lancet Psychiatry, 2*(8), 710–717.

Pearson, J., Naselaris, T., Holmes, E. A., & Kosslyn, S. M. (2015). Mental imagery: Functional mechanisms and clinical applications. *Trends in Cognitive Sciences, 19*(10), 590–602.

Perlis, R. H., Ostacher, M. J., Patel, J. K., Marangell, L. B., Zhang, H., Wisniewski, S. R., et al. (2006). Predictors of recurrence in bipolar disorder: Primary outcomes from the Systematic Treatment Enhancement Program for Bipolar Disorder (STEP-BD). *American Journal of Psychiatry, 163*(2), 217–224.

Perls, F. (1973). *The Gestalt approach and eye witness to therapy.* Palo Alto, CA: Science & Behavior Books.

Pratt, D., Cooper, M. J., & Hackmann, A. (2004). Imagery and its characteristics in people who are anxious about spiders. *Behavioural and Cognitive Psychotherapy, 32,* 165–176.

Rachman, S. (1980). Emotional processing. *Behaviour Research and Therapy, 18*(1), 51–60.

Rachman, S. (2001). Emotional processing, with special reference to post-traumatic stress disorders. *International Review of Psychiatry, 13*(3), 164–171.

Rademacher, J., DelBello, M. P., Adler, C., Stanford, K., & Strakowski, S. M. (2007). Health-related quality of life in adolescents with bipolar I disorder. *Journal of Child and Adolescent Psychopharmacology, 17*(1), 97–103.

Reisberg, D., Pearson, D. G., & Kosslyn, S. M. (2003). Intuitions and introspections about imagery: The role of imagery experience in shaping an investigator's theoretical views. *Applied Cognitive Psychology, 17*(2), 147–160.

Renner, F., Murphy, F., Ji, J., Manly, T., & Holmes, E. A. (2019). Mental imagery as a "motivational amplifier" to promote activities. *Behavior Research and Therapy, 11,* 51–59.

Rush, J. A., Trivedi, M. H., Ibrahim, H. M., Carmody, T. J., Arnow, B., Klein, D. N., et al. (2003). The 16-item Quick Inventory of Depressive Symptomatology (QIDS), Clinician Rating (QIDS-C), and Self-Report (QIDS-SR): A psychometric evaluation in patients with chronic major depression. *Biological Psychiatry, 54*(5), 573–583.

Scott, J. (2011). Bipolar disorder: From early identification to personalized treatment. *Early Intervention in Psychiatry, 5*(2), 89–90.

Scott, J., Paykel, E. S., Morriss, R., Kinderman, P., Johnson, T., Abbott, R., & Hayhurst, H. (2006). Cognitive-behavioural therapy for severe and recurrent bipolar disorders: Randomised controlled trial. *British Journal of Psychiatry, 188*(4), 313–320.

Scott, J., Stanton, B., Garland, A., & Ferrier, I. N. (2000). Cognitive vulnerability in patients with bipolar disorder. *Psychological Medicine, 30*(2), 467–472.

Shapiro, F. (2001). *Eye movement desensitization and reprocessing: Basic principles, protocols and procedures* (2nd ed.). New York: Guilford Press.

Shapiro, F. (2018). *Eye movement desensitization and reprocessing (EMDR) therapy: Basic principles, protocols, and procedures* (3rd ed.). New York: Guilford Press.

Simon, N. M., Otto, M. W., Wisniewski, S. R., Fossey, M., Sagduyu, K., Frank, E., et al. (2004). Anxiety disorder comorbidity in bipolar disorder patients: Data from the first 500 participants in the Systematic Treatment Enhancement Program for Bipolar Disorder (STEP-BD). *American Journal of Psychiatry, 161*(12), 2222–2229.

Simon, N. M., Pollack, M. H., Ostacher, M. J., Zalta, A. K., Chow, C. W., Fischmann, D., et al. (2007). Understanding the link between anxiety symptoms and suicidal ideation and behaviors in outpatients with bipolar disorder. *Journal of Affective Disorders, 97*(1–3), 91–99.

Skinner, B. F. (1953). *Science and human behavior.* New York: Macmillan.

Skjelstad, D. V., Malt, U. F., & Holte, A. (2010).

Symptoms and signs of the initial prodrome of bipolar disorder: A systematic review. *Journal of Affective Disorders, 126,* 1–13.

Smucker, M. R., Dancu, C. V., Foa, E. B., & Niederee, J. L. (1995). Imagery rescripting: A new treatment for survivors of childhood sexual abuse suffering from post-traumatic stress. *Journal of Cognitive Psychotherapy: An International Quarterly, 9,* 3–17.

Somerville, K., Cooper, M., & Hackmann, A. (2007). Spontaneous imagery in women with bulimia nervosa: An investigation into content, characteristics and links to childhood memories. *Journal of Behavior Therapy and Experimental Psychiatry, 38*(4), 435–446.

Stampfl, T. G., & Levis, D. J. (1967). Essentials of implosive therapy: A learning-theory-based psychodynamic behavioral therapy. *Journal of Abnormal Psychology, 72*(6), 496–503.

Steil, R., Jung, K., & Stangier, U. (2011). Efficacy of a two-session program of cognitive restructuring and imagery modification to reduce the feeling of being contaminated in adult survivors of childhood sexual abuse: A pilot study. *Journal of Behavior Therapy and Experimental Psychiatry, 42*(3), 325–329.

Stratford, H., Blackwell, S. E., Di Simplicio, M., Cooper, M., & Holmes, E. A. (2014). Psychological therapy for anxiety in bipolar spectrum disorders: A systematic review. *Clinical Psychological Review, 35,* 19–34.

Strejilevich, S. A., Martino, D. J., Murru, A, Teitelbaum, J., Fassi, G., Marengo, E., et al. (2013). Mood instability and functional recovery in bipolar disorders. *Acta Psychiatrica Scandinavica, 128*(3), 194–202.

van den Hout, M. A., & Engelhard, I. M. (2012). How does EMDR work? *Journal of Experimental Psychopathology, 3*(5), 724–738.

Walton, G. M., & Cohen, G. L. (2011). A brief social-belonging intervention improves academic and health outcomes of minority students. *Science, 331*(6023), 1447–1451.

Webb, R. T., Lichtenstein, P., Larsson, H., Geddes, J. R., & Fazel, S. (2014). Suicide, hospital-presenting suicide attempts, and criminality in bipolar disorder: Examination of risk for multiple adverse outcomes. *Journal of Clinical Psychiatry, 75*(8), e809–e816.

Weertman, A., & Arntz, A. (2007). Effectiveness of treatment of childhood memories in cognitive therapy for personality disorders: A controlled study contrasting methods focusing on the present and methods of focusing on childhood memories. *Behaviour Research and Therapy, 45,* 2133–2143.

Wegner, D. M., Schneider, D. J., Carter, S. R., & White, T. L. (1987). Paradoxical effects of thought suppression. *Journal of Personality and Social Psychology, 53,* 5–13.

Wells, A., & Clark, D. (1997). Social phobia: A cognitive approach. In G. C. L. Davey (Ed.), *Phobias: A handbook of theory, research and treatment* (pp. 3–26). Chichester, UK: Wiley.

Wheatley, J., Brewin, C. R., Patel, T., Hackmann, A., Wells, A., Fisher, P., et al. (2007). "I'll believe it when I can see it": Imagery rescripting of intrusive sensory memories in depression. *Journal of Behavior Therapy and Experimental Psychiatry, 38*(4), 371–385.

Wild, J., Hackmann, A., & Clark, D. M. (2007). When the present visits the past: Updating traumatic memories in social phobia. *Journal of Behavior Therapy and Experimental Psychiatry, 38*(4), 386–401.

Wild, J., Hackmann, A., & Clark, D. M. (2008). Rescripting early memories linked to negative images in social phobia: A pilot study. *Behavior Therapy, 39*(1), 47–56.

Wolpe, J. (1958). *Psychotherapy by reciprocal inhibition.* Stanford, CA: Stanford University Press.

Yatham, L. N., Kennedy, S. H., Parikh, S. V., Schaffer, A., Beaulieu, S., Alda, M., et al. (2013). Canadian Network for Mood and Anxiety Treatments (CANMAT) and International Society for Bipolar Disorders (ISBD) collaborative update of CANMAT guidelines for the management of patients with bipolar disorder: Update 2013. *Bipolar Disorder, 15*(1), 1–44.

Young, J. E., Klosko, J. S., & Weishaar, M. E. (2003). *Schema therapy: A practitioner's guide.* New York: Guilford Press.

Zaretsky, A., Lancee, W., Miller, C., Harris, A. J. L., & Parikh, S. V. (2008). Is cognitive-behavioural therapy more effective than psychoeducation in bipolar disorder? *Canadian Journal of Psychiatry, 53*(7), 441–448.

Index

Note. *f* or *t* following a page number indicates a figure or a table.